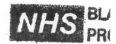 

NHS BL
PR(

D1418727

A Pocket Guide fc

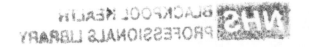

This second edition is dedicated to a group of students, September '05 intake, for whom we both had the privilege of being personal teacher at different times:

Caz, Charlotte, Helen, Leanne, Maggie, Michelle, Sarah J. and Sarah T.

Their motivation, hard work and commitment to midwifery resulted in high achievements academically and successful qualification and registration as midwives. Best wishes for your careers as midwives.

A Pocket Guide for Student Midwives

Second Edition

Stella McKay-Moffat
MPhil., BA (Hons) RN, RM, ADM, Cert. Ed.
Family Planning Certificate
Senior Lecturer Midwifery and Women's Health
Edge Hill University

Pam Lee
MA (Social policy), BA (Hons) RN, RM, MTD,
Dip. N (Lond.) FETC
Dip. Applied Social Sciences, ENB N07
Post Grad. Diploma in Psychosexual Therapy
Psychosexual Counsellor
Associate Lecturer Midwifery and Women's Health
Edge Hill University

WILEY-BLACKWELL
A John Wiley & Sons, Ltd., Publication

First edition published 2006
This edition first published 2010
© 2006, 2010 by John Wiley & Sons Ltd

Wiley-Blackwell is an imprint of John Wiley & Sons, formed by the merger of Wiley's global Scientific, Technical and Medical business with Blackwell Publishing.

Registered office: John Wiley & Sons Ltd, The Atrium, Southern Gate, Chichester, West Sussex, PO19 8SQ, United Kingdom

Editorial office: John Wiley & Sons Ltd, The Atrium, Southern Gate, Chichester, West Sussex, PO19 8SQ, United Kingdom

For details of our global editorial offices, for customer services and for information about how to apply for permission to reuse the copyright material in this book please see our website at www.wiley.com/wiley-blackwell.

The right of the author to be identified as the author of this work has been asserted in accordance with the UK Copyright, Designs and Patents Act 1988.

Library of Congress Cataloging-in-Publication Data
McKay-Moffat, Stella.
    A pocket guide for student midwives / Stella McKay-Moffat, Pam Lee. – 2nd ed.
        p. ; cm.
    Includes bibliographical references.
        ISBN 978-0-470-71243-6 (pbk. : alk. paper)   1.   Midwifery – Handbooks, manuals, etc.
I. Lee, Pamela, RN. II. Title.
    [DNLM: 1.   Midwifery – Handbooks.   WQ 165 M478p 2010]
    RG950.M43 2010
    618.2 – dc22

                                                                            2010004439

A catalogue record for this book is available from the British Library.

Typeset in 8/12 StoneSerif by Laserwords Private Limited, Chennai, India
Printed and bound in Singapore by Fabulous Printers Pte Ltd

1   2010

Contents

Contents

Contents

Contents

Contents

About the authors

Stella and Pam are very experienced midwives and midwifery lecturers, having taught a range of learners from pre-registration students to qualified staff. Both authors embrace innovation and advancement in the maternity services and midwifery profession, whilst valuing the quality of appropriate traditional practices.

Stella spent over 15 years in practice, with more than 11 of those in the community offering the whole range of maternity services, including home birth. She has a keen interest in women's health, and in particular, in contraception and family planning. Her M.Phil. research explored maternity services for women with disabilities and midwives' experiences of providing those services. Stella acts as an external examiner for Salford University for qualified midwives studying part-time for a midwifery degree.

Having gained an MA in Social Policy, Pam has a special interest in the social policy-making process, particularly in relation to the maternity services. Another area of her interest and expertise is around sexuality and body image. Pam is a qualified psychosexual therapist practising within the women's sexual health services of a local trust. Since retiring from her full-time post as senior lecturer, Pam continues as a valued associate lecturer.

Preface

The first edition of this book was inspired by comments from student midwives in the authors' educational institution. They said, 'We need something to help us survive the midwifery course'. Both authors are aware of students' anxieties and frustration at the vast amount of information and skills that have to be learned to become a midwife. Positive and constructive feedback from students using the first edition and a rapidly changing maternity service have prompted the production of this updated edition.

Midwifery is a practice-based profession that is both an art and a science. There are frequently many different ways of achieving the same satisfactory learning outcome; the lack of 'black and white' or 'hard and fast' rules in the majority of the elements of the profession may make learning difficult to cope with. This is particularly noticeable as practitioners are striving, in line with government directives in the *Maternity Standards of the National Service Framework* (NSF) (DH 2004) and *Maternity Matters* (DH 2007a), to facilitate a high-quality service that meets the needs of women and their partners in the twenty-first century. However, students should take heart that once the 'basics' of a situation have been learnt, the 'variations' can be added to the repertoire of knowledge and skills.

Practice needs to be underpinned by a sound theoretical framework that is evidence based. In an endeavour to help students grasp the appropriate knowledge and understanding, link theory to practice and 'survive the midwifery course', the present pocket book has been written to provide quick, easy-to-read information and guidelines on the 'basics' in midwifery that could be taken on duty. The instant access to information will provide some theory, trigger thought and give directions to support practice in an easily repeatable process.

Student midwives who are already registered nurses may find that some of the basic nursing procedures are already within their capabilities. Nevertheless, revision is often useful, and some procedures may, in fact, have a different focus, as they are centred on the (generally) healthy childbearing woman rather than the sick patient.

The book is in two sections, each arranged alphabetically. The first section contains some of the language of midwifery: terms, abbreviations and definitions. A few terms are colloquial and not necessarily 'medically' correct but are included, however, to enable clarification of understanding and to prompt the use of correct terminology. The second section contains common conditions, procedures, emergency situations and supporting information. Where conditions are noted the aetiology is given, if known. Each topic may include further factors that involve recognition, prevention and actions to be taken in an emergency situation that may be in the form of flow/action charts. These action charts should be read from top left. The flow lines are followed depending on the circumstances at the time. The procedures that are included have an overview of the 'how to' (frequently including the preparation needed) and the 'why' supported by research or evidence, and *Midwives' Rules and Standards* (Nurses and Midwives Council (NMC) 2004) and The NMC *Code of Professional Conduct: Standards for Conduct, Performance and Ethics (The Code)* (NMC 2008). The references used could provide useful evidence to support practice. Finally, the supporting information is varied, and ranges from details about government and international initiatives to available support groups and useful websites.

As no topic is in isolation, many categories are cross-referenced and extra reading/activities are suggested to enhance the reader's knowledge. Furthermore, additional study may be needed to understand and learn the anatomy, the physiology and possibly the biochemistry associated with the conditions included.

Finally, the authors appreciate that local policies and protocols vary; therefore, the reader is recommended to consider topics in the light of those local guidelines as well as of the emergence of new evidence that informs practice.

Acknowledgements

We would like to thank Lawrence Berry, Media Resources Officer at Edge Hill University, for his help and expertise in producing the graphics for the original edition, and Carol Revill-Johnson, Senior Midwifery Lecturer and Advanced Life Support in Obstetrics trainer, for her constructive criticism ensuring the charts reflect current guidelines.

Section 1

The language of midwifery

In a new environment, one key to understanding is to have knowledge of the language that is used. To this end, this section contains an alphabetical list of terms, abbreviations and definitions frequently used in midwifery, nursing and medicine. Terms in italics may be heard of but are colloquial; however, they are included here not only to help in the understanding of the 'everyday' language used but also to encourage the use of correct terminology.

Symbols are frequently used as a form of 'shorthand' in clinical practice, therefore some commonly used ones are included at the beginning of this section of the book to enhance understanding. Some may be used throughout the book.

$\cong$ approximate	$\leq$ less than or equal to
$\geq$ more than or equal to	Δ diagnosis
$\uparrow$ raised/increased	$\downarrow$ lowered/decreased
$<$ less than/before	$>$ greater than/after
R_x prescribe/prescription	# fracture(d) (usually bone)
? query, question, possible	μmol/l micromol per litre

A Pocket Guide for Student Midwives: Second edition, by Stella McKay-Moffat and Pam Lee. © 2010 by John Wiley & Sons Ltd.

ABO blood groups – classification system according to the presence of antigens on red blood cells/antibodies in serum (see also **Rhesus factor**)

Blood group	Antigen on cell	Antibody in serum
O	none	anti-A and anti-B
A	A	anti-B
B	B	anti-A
AB	A and B	none

blood group O Rh negative = universal donor (can give to any group in an emergency)
blood group AB Rh positive = universal recipient (can receive from any group in an emergency)
Abortion – expulsion of the products of conception from the uterus <24th week of gestation – can be induced (termination) or spontaneous (miscarriage – see subsequent entry)
Acceleration/active phase of cervical dilatation – more rapid cervical dilatation after 5 cm – recorded on a partogram (approximately 1 cm per hour)
Acceleration/augmentation of labour – process by which spontaneous labour is made more efficient through intervention
Accountability – liability to be called to account for one's conduct; responsibility for practising professionally
Active birth – one in which the woman participates fully in her labour, is totally aware of what is going on in her body and is able to respond naturally
Active management of labour – assessing/monitoring progress and implementing policies to prevent prolonged labour (see **Acceleration/augmentation of labour**)
Adoption – a formal legal procedure that severs the relationship between a child and its parent(s) and establishes a new one with its adoptive parents
Adoption agency/society – a local authority (LA) or voluntary organisation whose function consists of or includes making arrangements for the adoption of children. Voluntary agencies must be registered with the LA and be open to inspection, and are non-profit-making, but may charge fees for services provided

AFE – amniotic fluid embolism – see Section 2

AFP – **alpha fetoprotein** – a precursor to plasma protein produced by the fetus and excreted into the amniotic fluid. High levels of AFP in maternal blood can be used as part of a risk assessment for fetal neural tube defects and low levels for Down's syndrome. Prenatal diagnosis of neural tube defects is effected by assessing AFP in the liquor following amniocentesis

Alternative birth positions – positions other than the dorsal position that the mother may choose when giving birth, e.g. a squatting position, an upright position, a kneeling position

Amnion – a tough, smooth, translucent membrane derived from the inner cell mass of the embryo. It lines the chorion and covers the fetal surface of the placenta as far as the insertion of the umbilical cord. It contains the amniotic fluid (liquor) and contributes to its formation

Amniotomy – rupturing the forewaters – see **ARM, Acceleration/ augmentation of labour**

AN – **antenatal(ly)**

Anaesthesia – loss of sensation induced by anaesthetic agents to allow surgery – total/partial anaesthesia, with/without loss of consciousness

Analgesia – insensibility to pain without loss of consciousness, i.e. pain relief

Antepartum haemorrhage (APH) – bleeding from the genital tract >24 weeks of pregnancy

Anti-D immunoglobulin – a blood product given IM to Rhesus-negative women to prevent isoimmunisation to the D part of the Rhesus factor (see **Rhesus factor**)

Apgar score – a scoring system devised by Dr Virginia Apgar in 1958 to assess the newborn's condition for resuscitation purposes (see **Delivery technique**, Delivery of head in occipito-anterior position in Section 2)

APH – **antepartum haemorrhage** – bleeding from the genital tract >24 weeks of pregnancy

APTT – **activated partial thromboplastin time** – a blood test related to the clotting mechanism – normal clotting time approximately 25–35 seconds

ARDS – **adult/acute respiratory distress syndrome** (see **RDS**)

ARM – artificial rupture of membranes – manually perforating the bag of forewaters containing the fetus (see Section 2 and **Acceleration/augmentation of labour**)

AST – aspartate aminotransferase – an enzyme that catalyses salts of the amino acid aspartamine – blood levels raised with liver/heart damaged (see **PIH** and **Pre-eclampsia** in Sections 1 and 2)

Attitude – relationship of fetal head and limbs to the trunk, e.g. flexion, deflexion (often called a military attitude), partial extension and full extension

Baby – the fetus when completely expelled from the uterus >24 weeks gestation

Baby blues – third/fourth day blues – feeling emotionally low following childbirth (see **Postnatal depression** in Section 2)

Bandl's ring – an exaggerated retraction ring that occurs when labour is obstructed – ? palpated abdominally, and is a serious sign (see **Retraction ring**)

Barlow's test – screening test for CDH, modified from Ortolani's test

Battledore insertion – cord inserted at the very edge of the placenta (see **Placental examination** in Section 2)

BBA – born before arrival – baby born before arrival of midwife/doctor

BD/bid (*bis in die*) – twice daily – often on a prescription

BF – breastfeeding

BFI – Breastfeeding Initiative or Baby Friendly Initiative (see Section 2)

Biophysical profile – assessment of the fetal condition using indicators such as fetal breathing movements, Doppler techniques, amniotic fluid measurement

Bipartite/tripartite placenta – one divided into two or three distinct areas (see **Placental examination** in Section 2)

Bishop's score – method of assessing the suitability of the cervix for induction of labour by noting the length and softness and dilatation of the cervical os (opening)

Blades – obstetric forceps

BLS – basic life support (see **Birth asphyxia and BLS – adult** in Section 2)

BM sticks/test – originally a colour-changing reagent strip for measuring peripheral blood glucose made by Boehringer Mannheim. Term often used colloquially for all estimations of peripheral blood glucose. Modern sticks from various makers are used with an electrical–optical measuring device for greater accuracy

BMI – body mass index – indicator of ideal weight, obesity or underweight. Calculation: weight in kilograms is divided by square of height in metres (weight [kg]/height [m^2]) – undertaken at antenatal booking interview (see **Obesity in pregnancy** in Section 2)

BO – bowels opened – faeces passed

Bradycardia – slowing of the heart rate: in adults <60 beats per minute and in fetus <100 beats per minute

Brandt–Andrews – method of delivering the placenta without oxytocic drugs (see **Delivery technique**, Third-stage management in Section 2)

Braxton Hicks contractions – painless uterine contractions, part of the physiological growth/stretching process during pregnancy

Breech – the lower fetal pole, including buttocks and legs (see **Presentation** and **Breech delivery** in Section 2)

Brim of the pelvis – bony ring formed by the following landmarks (posteriorly to anteriorly): sacral promontory, sacral ala or wing, sacroiliac joint, iliopectineal line, iliopectineal eminence, superior ramus of the pubic bone, upper inner body of the pubic bone and the symphysis pubis, continuing round in a circle

Brow – area on fetal skull from supra-orbital ridges to coronal suture (see **Presentation** and **Occipito-posterior position** in Section 2)

Buttonholing – of perineum, i.e. as the perineum is distending during advancement of the fetal head, small areas of tissue begin to separate, causing an opening

C & S – culture and sensitivity – request on a form sent to laboratory with a specimen, e.g. MSSU, HVS – for culture (growth and identification of the organism) and testing its sensitivity (to antibiotics that may be used against it)

Caput succedaneum – soft swelling because of fluid (oedema) on the fetal scalp due to pressure on the head during labour (can cross a suture line of the skull bones – compare with cephalhaematoma)

CCT – controlled cord traction (see **Delivery technique**, Third-stage management in Section 2)

CDH – congenital dislocation of the hip

CEMACH – Confidential Enquiry into Maternal and Child Health (see Section 2 and **Maternal mortality rate**)

Ceph/cephalic – pertaining to the fetal head (see **Presentation**)

Cephalhaematoma – swelling on newborn's head due to bleeding beneath the periosteum associated with traumatic delivery (does not cross a suture line of the skull – compare with **caput succedaneum**)

Cephalo-pelvic disproportion (CPD) – fetal head will not pass through the maternal pelvis (see Section 2)

Cervix – the lower one-third of the uterus

CESDI – Confidential Enquiry into Stillbirth and Deaths in Infancy (see Section 2 and **CEMACH**)

Chasing the dragon – smoking heroin (diamorphine) by lighting the powder on aluminium foil and inhaling the fumes

CF – cystic fibrosis (see **Heel prick** and **Neonatal screening** in Section 2)

Chignon – swelling on newborn's head following vacuum extraction (see **Instrumental delivery** in Section 2) as soft tissues are drawn into the cup during the procedure (compare with **caput succedaneum and cephalhaematoma**)

Chorion – a thick, opaque, friable membrane that develops from the trophoblast. It is continuous with the edge of the placenta, lines the **amnion** and is closely adherent to the **decidua**

CHT – congenital hypothyroidism (see **Hypothyroidism** in Section 2)

CIN – cervical intra-epithelial neoplasm – early cervical cell changes that could progress to cancer if not treated

Circumvallate placenta – one with a double fold of chorion round the edge of the placenta, causing a ridge (see **Placental examination** in Section 2)

CONI – care of next infant (see **Sudden infant death syndrome** in Section 2)

Confidentiality – a trusting relationship in which secrets may be imparted – the midwife has a duty to respect confidentiality except where disclosure is required by law (see *The Code: Standards of Conduct, Performance and Ethics for Nurses and Midwives* (NMC 2008))

Coombs test – performed on cord blood to detect maternal antibodies on fetal red cells (see **Rhesus factor**)

Cotyledon – a clump of chorionic villi surrounded by maternal blood: 10–30 of them form the maternal surface of the placenta, i.e. the surface attached to the uterus (see **Placental examination** in Section 2)

CPD – cephalo-pelvic disproportion (see **Prolonged labour** in Sections 1 and 2)

CPR – cardiopulmonary resuscitation

Cracking on – labour is progressing, often rapidly

Crash bleep – emergency bleep – method of urgently summoning aid (usually medical) – familiarise yourself with your unit's protocol

Cricoid pressure – occlusion of the oesophagus by pressure applied to the cricoid cartilage (i.e. Sellick's manoeuvre) to prevent inhalation of reflux of stomach content during initiation of anaesthetic and before an endotracheal tube (ET) is inserted to maintain the airway

CSF – cerebrospinal fluid

CT/CAT scan – computerised (computer-assisted) tomography – computers record body 'slices' from X-ray scan pictures

CTG – cardiotocograph

Curve of Carus – an arc from the pelvic brim to the pelvic outlet, i.e. through the true pelvis, which the baby passes through during labour and birth

CVP – central venous pressure – right atrium blood pressure; indicates circulatory function/blood volume, especially in shock/during blood replacement

Cystic fibrosis (CF) – A congenital condition caused by a recessive gene present in 1:25 people in the United Kingdom leading to 1:2000 babies with the condition. The disorder leads to thick, sticky mucus production with poor intestinal absorption, repeated chest infections and chronic lung disease. Abnormal sweat and saliva secretion is present.

Decidua – thickened endometrium (uterine lining) during pregnancy
Denominator – a fixed point on the presenting part determining the fetal position
Diabetes mellitus – a disorder of carbohydrate metabolism; insufficient insulin production/inability of cell response to insulin, resulting in high blood glucose levels; may occur in pregnancy without any previous history (gestational diabetes)
Diameter – a measurement from one point to another through the pelvis or the fetal skull
DIC – **disseminated intravascular coagulation** (coagulopathy) – specific conditions (e.g. haemorrhage, pre-eclampsia) result in excessive use of clotting factors, leading to bleeding that is difficult to control
Dips – falls in fetal heart rate – correct terminology is decelerations
Directed pushing – instructing the mother to bear down with each contraction (see **Valsalva manoeuvre**)
Dirty Duncan – see **Matthews Duncan**
Dizygotic – developing from two ova and sperms (see **Multiple pregnancy** in Sections 1 and 2)
DTA – deep transverse arrest – the baby's head has become lodged in the pelvis in the transverse diameter, needing rotation with forceps or delivery by caesarean section
Dubowitz score – system for assessing baby's gestational age: initially using 10 neurological and 11 physical criteria (Dubowitz *et al.* 1970); later modified (Dubowitz *et al.* 1998)
DVT – deep vein thrombosis (blood clot) – commonly found in a calf vein

Eclampsia – serious pregnancy complication where eclamptic convulsions occur – usually follows fulminating pre-eclampsia, possibly without previous signs/symptoms, especially postnatally
ECV – external cephalic version
EDD/EDC/EDB – estimated/expected date of delivery/confinement/birth – developed in 1912 by a German physician, Naegele's rule calculates due date by adding 7 days and 9 months to first day (of bleeding) of last menstrual period (LMP) – accuracy challenged; see Olsen (1999)

Edinburgh postnatal depression score – a questionnaire designed to help predict which women may be at risk of postnatal depression

Embryo – the developing conceptus from the third to the eighth week following fertilisation

Engagement of the fetal head – when the widest part of the head passes through the pelvic brim (usually the biparietal diameter)

Epidural block – a method of giving analgesia/anaesthesia by putting a local anaesthetic agent into the epidural space

Ergometrine – an oxytocic agent with a sustained uterine action; takes 6–7 minutes to act when given IM (0.5 mg); can also be given IV; acts within 45 seconds (0.25 mg)

ESR – erythrocyte sedimentation rate – measures the distance (in millimetres) at which red blood cells settle towards the bottom of a specially marked test tube in unclotted blood over the course of an hour. Useful in detecting and monitoring infection, including tuberculosis, tissue necrosis and rheumatism and arthritis

ET tube – endotracheal tube – tube passed into trachea to maintain an open airway; has an outer cuff that is inflated with air to make a seal

EWS/MEWS/MOEWS – early/modified early/modified obstetric early warning system – close monitoring of an individual's mental responses; vital signs (pulse, systolic BP, respirations [often the best early warning sign], temperature); urine output to detect early indications of deterioration in condition enabling rapid response/reduction in morbidity and mortality

Face – area on fetal skull from where the head joins the neck to the coronal suture and anterior fontanelle (see **Presentation** and **Delivery technique** in Section 2)

Fallot's tetralogy – cardiac abnormality causing cyanotic heart disease: comprises pulmonary stenosis, overriding aorta, ventricular septal defect and right ventricular hypertrophy

FBC – full blood count – numbers of all types of cells; often on a laboratory request form

Fetal distress – the fetus is compromised, suffering oxygen deprivation, becoming hypoxic (see **Birth asphyxia** in Section 2)

Fetus – the developing conceptus from the embryo (first to eighth weeks) until birth, when it becomes a neonate

FH, FHH or FHHR – fetal heart, fetal heart heard/heard and regular

First degree tear – involves the vaginal mucosa and/or the skin of the perineum, but not muscle

Flat baby (not an acceptable term) – asphyxiated baby (see **Birth asphyxia** in Section 2)

FM/FMF – fetal movements/movements felt

Folic acid – a member of the vitamin B complex, occurring in green plants, fresh fruits, liver and yeast; necessary for normal fetal CNS development; advised as a supplement pre-conception and in early pregnancy (see **Neural tube defect** in Section 2)

Fontanelle – membranous space on baby's skull where two or more suture lines meet (see **Vaginal examination** in Section 2)

Forewaters – amniotic fluid trapped before the fetal head as labour progresses (see **ARM** and **Vaginal examination** in Section 2)

Fourchette – a fold of skin between the vaginal entrance and the perineum

FSE – fetal scalp electrode – for continuous electronic monitoring of FH (see **CTG**)

Full dilatation of the cervix – when no cervix is felt on vaginal examination; uterine opening is approximately 10 cm

Fundus – upper part of the uterus between the areas of Fallopian tube insertion (the cornua)

GA – general anaesthetic

Gas and air – gaseous mixture of 50% oxygen/50% nitrous oxide (Entonox) inhaled for analgesia during labour

Gas man – nickname for an anaesthetist

Gestation – gestational age, i.e. pregnancy/weeks of pregnancy. Length of pregnancy is 280 days from LMP or 266 days from conception – it is not always clear which calculation is being used

Glabella – the bridge of the nose; glabellar tap – primitive reflex elicited in the newborn (see **Initial newborn examination** in Section 2)

Gown up – dressing in a sterile gown (frequently green) – prior to aseptic/sterile technique, ensuring gown sterility is not broken

Gravid – pregnant; hence gravidity (number of times pregnant), primigravida, multigravida

GTT – glucose tolerance test (see also **OGTT**)

Guthrie test – phenylketonuria screening 8–10 days following birth; microbiological techniques are used on filter paper soaked with blood; seldom used now (see also **Scriver test** and **Heel prick** in Section 2)

Haemorrhoids – varicose veins of the rectum/anus common in pregnancy owing to the effects of progesterone (see **Varicose veins** in Section 2)

Haemorrhage – excessive blood loss leading to shock (see **Antepartum** and **Post-partum haemorrhage** in Sections 1 and 2)

Hb – haemoglobin – blood level routinely screened for (see **Anaemia** in Section 2)

HV – health visitor

HVS – high vaginal swab – infection screening

Hydatidiform mole – gestational trophoblastic disease, usually without development of the fetus. Long-term follow-up required after evacuation of uterus due to risk of chorionic carcinoma

Hypertension – abnormally high arterial blood pressure; a diastolic blood pressure of 90 mmHg is significantly high in pregnancy (see **Pregnancy-induced hypertension and pre-eclampsia** in Section 2)

Hypoglycaemia – reduction in blood glucose levels; normal fasting blood glucose is 3–5 mmol/l (adult), less in the neonate (see **Heel prick** in Section 2)

Hypothermia – reduction in body temperature; below 35°C in the neonate (see **Temperature taking** in Section 2)

Hypothyroidism – reduced production of thyroid hormone from the thyroid gland; congenital or acquired (see **Hypothyroidism, Heel prick** and **Neonatal screening** in Section 2)

ICU – intensive care unit

IDD/IDDM – insulin-dependent diabetes/insulin-dependent diabetes mellitus

IM – intramuscular – an injection into a muscle (see **Administration of drugs** in Section 2)

Induction of labour – initiation of labour by artificial means

Infant – baby from birth to the end of the first year

Infant mortality rate – number of babies dying annually during the first year of life per 1000 live births. Rate 5.0 in England and Wales in 2006 (Norman *et al.* 2008); 4.6 in England and Wales in 2008 (Office for National Statistics 2010)

INR – international normalised ratio – a blood test measuring the ratios of clotting factors as part of the clotting mechanism screening

Insulin – hormone produced by the islets of Langerhans in the pancreas; a transport mechanism for glucose/regulates carbohydrate metabolism; given synthetically in diabetes mellitus

Intrapartum – during birth (second stage of labour)

Intrauterine growth restriction (*retardation*) (IUGR) – fetal growth falling below that expected, when the birth weight is below the tenth centile for gestational age (see **Intrauterine growth restriction** and **Small-for-gestational-age babies** in Section 2)

Intubation – passage of an endotracheal (ET) tube into the trachea for resuscitation purposes and to maintain a clear airway

Involution of the uterus – the process by which the uterus shrinks to (almost) its pre-pregnant shape, size and situation; brought about by autolysis and phagocytosis

IUCD/IUD – intrauterine contraceptive device (coil) – beware of next abbreviation

IUD – intrauterine death (note earlier abbreviation)

IUGR – intrauterine growth restriction (*retardation*) (see earlier entry and Section 2)

IV – intravenous – usually an injection/infusion (see **Administration of drugs** in Section 2)

IVI – intravenous infusion

Jaundice – yellow skin/mucous membrane discoloration when serum bilirubin levels reach 80 µmol/l

Karyotype – a visual arrangement of all chromosomes from a single cell, enabling identification/counting

Kernicterus – staining of the basal ganglia in the brain due to high levels of unconjugated (fat-soluble) bilirubin; causes severe damage, including blindness, deafness and cerebral palsy (see **Jaundice** in Section 2)

Ketoacidosis – metabolic disorder resulting from insufficient carbohydrate intake; fats are metabolised instead, and ketone bodies formed (see **Diabetes mellitus**)

Kleihauer test – blood test on Rhesus-negative women estimating the number of fetal blood cells in maternal circulation following delivery; if large numbers ? extra anti-D immunoglobulin needed

Labour – a continuous physiological process of contraction and retraction (shortening) of the myometrium (uterine muscle) during which the products of conception are expelled from the uterus

1. First stage – sometimes considered to be in three phases, although demarcation is imprecise and there is no professional consensus

Latent phase – (equates to the lay definition of 'slow labour') the early preparation stage, lasting hours or days. Contractions may be regular or irregular, frequent or intermittent, painful or painless, weak or fairly strong. The cervix effaces (shortens) and slowly dilates from closed (in primigravida) or slightly open, i.e. multips os (in multigravida), up to approximately 4 cm dilated.

Active or acceleration phase – a continuation of the latent phase, i.e. now established labour. Contractions become progressively more regular, frequent, strong and painful. Cervical dilatation progresses at approximately 1 cm per hour to full dilatation (about 10 cm), and the presenting part (the fetal head in normal labour) progresses through the maternal pelvis.

Deceleration phase – progress of cervical dilatation from 9 to 10 cm is sometimes delayed as contractions briefly fade (mother and uterus 'rest') before full dilatation is achieved – causes no concern unless there is fetal or maternal compromise.

2. Second stage – from full dilatation of the cervix to expulsion of the baby. The mother may not immediately have the urge to bear

Tv07852

down (push); await spontaneous expulsive effort (pushing), which is less traumatic for mother and baby than directed pushing (see **Valsalva manoeuvre**) unless there are signs of fetal compromise. Some mothers do need guidance and encouragement on pushing.

3. Third stage – from the birth of the baby until complete expulsion of placenta and membranes and the control of haemorrhage

Lanugo – fine, downy-like hair on the fetal body; some often remains at birth

Last menstrual period (LMP) – the first day of bleeding in a normal menstrual cycle; used to calculate the expected date of delivery/birth (EDD/B). Accuracy of this date is questionable because of variable menstrual cycles and ovulation dates

Latent phase of cervical dilatation – slow dilatation of the cervix up to approximately 4 cm (see earlier entry), seen especially in the primigravida; recorded on the partogram

Lecithin/sphingomyelin (LS) ratio – a test (less often performed now) on amniotic fluid to determine fetal lung maturity; should be greater than 2:1 (see **Antenatal screening** in Section 2); used as an indicator of lung surfactant levels and therefore lung maturity. A lower ratio indicates the potential for neonatal respiratory distress syndrome (surfactant deficiency syndrome SDS)

Lie – the relationship of the long axis of the fetus (fetal spine) to the long axis of the mother's uterus – usually longitudinal – may be oblique, transverse, unstable (see **Abdominal palpation** in Section 2)

Live birth – any baby born that breathes, cries or shows signs of life

LMP – Last menstrual period (see earlier entry)

Lochia – the discharges from the uterus following delivery – initially rubra (red) to serosa (red/brown) and then albicans (pale); noted in mother's records

LS ratio – the lecithin–sphingomyelin ratio (see earlier entry)

Malposition – where the occiput is posterior in the pelvis rather than the normal anterior

Malpresentation – where the fetal part lying lowest in the birth canal is not the normal vertex – i.e. face, brow, shoulder, breech, or compound presentation, e.g. head and hand

Maternal mortality rate – number of women dying during pregnancy, labour or within 42 days of giving birth, miscarriage or abortion per 100,000 maternities (i.e. known pregnancies). Direct death rate (i.e. caused by pregnancy) is 6.24 in the United Kingdom, with thromboembolic conditions remaining the lead cause (Lewis 2007 – see **Confidential Enquiry into Maternal and Child Health (CEMACH)** in Section 2)

Matthews Duncan – method of placental separation; the placenta is lying in the lower uterus and 'slides' off the wall, the maternal surface of the placenta appears at the vulva, often associated with excessive blood loss (the so-called *dirty Duncan*); compare with the Schultz method

(MCADD) – medium chain acyl-CoA dehydrogenase deficiency (see subsequent entry)

MCH – mean corpuscular haemoglobin (reported on blood test) – average amount of haemoglobin in the red blood cells (see **Anaemia** in Section 2)

MCV – mean corpuscular volume (reported on blood test) – average volume of a single red blood cell in cubic micrometres (μm^3), normally 90 (see **Anaemia** in Section 2)

Mechanism of labour – means by which the fetus negotiates the birth canal

Meconium (mec.) – greenish black substance present in fetal intestine/passed during the first 2–3 days of life. Contains bile salts and pigments, fetal cells and mucus. May be passed *in utero*; fresh/old meconium in liquor indicates how recently passed – may indicate fetal hypoxia or post maturity (see **Fetal distress** in Section 2)

Medium chain acyl-CoA dehydrogenase deficiency (MCADD) – autosomal recessive inherited disorder (i.e. both parents carry an affected gene) (see **Heel prick** and **Neonatal screening** in Section 2)

Mentum – chin – the denominator in a face presentation (see **Presentation**)

MEWS/MOEWS – see **EWS**

Miscarriage – loss of fetus <24 weeks gestation; a less emotive term to use with women than spontaneous abortion. May be total (complete abortion), partial (incomplete abortion) or retained (missed abortion)

Monozygotic – developing from one ovum and sperm (see **Dizygotic** and **Multiple pregnancy**)

Morbidity – state of ill health/disease; case numbers of a particular disease in a given population; commonly related to maternal/perinatal mortality

Mortality/mortality rate – death; the frequency/number of deaths in a given population (see **Infant mortality, Maternal mortality, Neonatal mortality, Perinatal mortality**, and **Stillbirth**)

Moulding – alteration in the shape of fetal skull allowing passage through the true pelvis; engaging diameter is reduced at the expense of the diameter 90° to it

MRI scan – magnetic resonance imaging scan – computers used to map variations in body tissue subjected to high-frequency radio waves, particularly useful for examining the central nervous system

MSSU/MSU – midstream specimen of urine (see **UTI** in Section 2)

Multigravida – a woman pregnant for the second or subsequent time (even if the previous pregnancy/ies resulted in miscarriage) – a grand(e) multigravida is a woman pregnant for a fifth or subsequent time

Multips os – the state of cervical os (opening), often used to mean the cervix itself, i.e. cervix not showing any indications that the woman is in labour, only that she has previously had a baby

Multiple pregnancy – simultaneous presence of more then one fetus

NAD – nothing abnormal discovered – commonly referring to results of a standard dipstick urine test, ? other examinations

NCT – National Childbirth Trust (see Section 2)

Neonate/neonatal – Baby up to 28 days old/pertaining to the first 28 days of life

Neonatal mortality rate (NMR) – number of neonates dying per 1000 live births annually. Rate was 3.4 in the United Kingdom in 2006 (CEMACH 2008); 3.2 in England and Wales in 2008 (Office for National Statistics 2010)

Neonatal screening – see Section 2

Niggler/niggling – a woman in spurious labour, i.e. having contractions in latent first stage but not in established labour

NNU/NNICU – neonatal unit/neonatal intensive care unit

Nocte – at night – often on a prescription

NTD – neural tube defect, e.g. spina bifida

OA – occipito-anterior, i.e. the occiput (back of fetal head) is in the anterior part of the maternal pelvis; direct OA, behind symphysis pubis; LOA or ROA, to left or right of symphysis pubis

Obs. or doing the Obs., i.e. observations; noting vital signs, e.g. temperature, pulse, blood pressure, respirations, ? others – e.g. fluid balance, level of consciousness

Obstetric forceps – two-bladed stainless steel instruments (see **Instrumental delivery** in Section 2)

Obstructed labour – no advance of presenting part despite good uterine contractions (see **Prolonged labour**)

Occiput – occipital bone of fetal skull – denominator in vertex presentation (see **Presentation**)

ODP/ODA/ODO – operating department practitioner/assistant/orderly – assists the anaesthetist

OES – obstetric emergency service/*flying squad* – deployed for community obstetric emergencies before paramedics became more skilled/available

OGGT – oral glucose tolerance test (see also **GTT** and **Diabetes**)

Oligohydramnios – reduced amniotic fluid (see Section 2)

OP position – occipito-posterior position, i.e. fetal occiput (back of head) in posterior part of maternal pelvis; direct OP, occiput in mother's sacrum; LOP or ROP, left or right of sacrum

Ophthalmia neonatorum – purulent eye discharge of the newborn occurring within 21 days of birth; no longer a notifiable disease; ? caused by *Gonococcus* organism/*Chlamydia trachomatis*

Ortolani's test – screening method for congenital dislocation of the hip, modified by Barlow

Oxytocic drugs – synthetic drugs mimicking the action of oxytocin from the posterior pituitary gland and causing uterine contractions (ergometrine, Syntometrine, Syntocinon)

Paed. – short for paediatrician

Parity – number of pregnancies >24 weeks, hence para 1, 2, multipara, grand(e) multipara (>4 babies)

Partogram/partograph – a chart for graphically entering the salient features of labour – progress represented visually, allowing easy recognition of deviations from normal

Parturition – childbirth; parity

Pelvimetry – accurate measurement of true pelvis performed by X-ray, carried out if cephalo-pelvic disproportion (CPD) is suspected

Perinatal – period before birth, at birth and up to 1 week following birth

Perinatal death – baby dies before, during or within 1 week of birth, i.e. stillbirth or early neonatal death

Perinatal mortality rate – number of perinatal deaths per 1000 total births (i.e. all stillbirths and live births) annually. Rate was 7.9 in the United Kingdom in 2006 (CEMACH 2008); 7.5 in England and Wales in 2008 (Office for National Statistics 2010)

PET – *Pre-eclamptic toxaemia* – no longer an accepted term (see **Pregnancy-induced hypertension/Pre-eclampsia** in Section 2)

PIH – pregnancy-induced hypertension

Pinard – fetal stethoscope; invented by French obstetrician Adolphe Pinard (1844–1934)

PKU – phenylketonuria – inborn error of metabolism (see Section 2)

PN – postnatal(ly)

Polyhydramnios – excess amniotic fluid

Position – relationship of denominator to a fixed point on the pelvis, e.g. right occipito-anterior (ROA) (see **Abdominal palpation** in Section 2)

Postmaturity/post-term – pregnancy >42 completed weeks; baby born after this period

Postnatal period – 'means the period after the end of labour during which the attendance of a midwife upon a woman and baby is required, being not less than 10 days and for such longer period as the midwife considers necessary' (NMC 2004, *Midwives' Rules and Standards*, p. 7)

Postneonatal – period from the end of the neonatal period until the end of the first year

PPH – postpartum haemorrhage – bleeding from the genital tract following the birth of the baby – 500 ml, or less if the woman is shocked; primary PPH, during the first 24 hours; secondary, after this; often 7–14 days (see Section 2)

Precipitate labour – sudden onset of labour/rapid delivery of baby

Pre-eclampsia – signs/symptoms possibly leading to eclampsia; fulminating pre-eclampsia, severe condition/imminent eclampsia (see **Pregnancy-induced hypertension/pre-eclampsia** in Section 2)

Premature rupture of membranes (PROM) – when the membranes rupture spontaneously 1 hour or more prior to the onset of labour (see Section 2)

Prematurity/preterm – where the pregnancy <37 completed weeks; labour which commences during this time; the resulting baby

Presentation/presenting part – the fetal part lying lowest in the birth canal – felt on abdominal palpation – usually the head (see **Abdominal palpation** in Section 2)

Primigravida – a woman pregnant for the first time

prn – (***pro re nata***) as required/indicated – often on prescription

Prolonged labour – lasting longer than expected; previously labour lasting >24 hours in a primigravida but this is now controversial as progress is the main consideration (see **Labour** in this section and **Prolonged labour – first stage** and **Prolonged labour – second stage** in Section 2)

PROM (Premature rupture of membranes) – when the membranes rupture spontaneously 1 hour prior to the onset of labour or earlier

PU – passing/passed urine

Puerperium – a 6-week period following the birth of the baby when the pelvic organs return to approximately their original size, shape and site and lactation is established

PV – *per vaginam* – examination, i.e. vaginal examination; or something passed, e.g. blood

Pyrexia – body temperature above 37°C; hyperpyrexia >40°C (see **Temperature-taking** in Section 2)

QDS/qid *(quarter in die)* – four times daily – often on a prescription

RDS – respiratory distress syndrome (surfactant deficiency syndrome SDS)

***Reg.* – registrar/senior registrar**, experienced senior doctor

Restitution – where the fetal head corrects itself to be aligned with the fetal back during the mechanism of labour

Retained placenta – failed delivery of placenta during third stage of labour – may/may not be wholly or partially separated from uterine wall

Retained products of conception – where products of conception remain in the uterus following miscarriage/birth; may lead to primary/secondary PPH

Retinopathy – condition associated with prematurity and diabetes; increased vascularisation behind the retina, leading to retinal damage and subsequent visual impairment in varying degrees

Retraction ring – occurs in normal labour at the junction of upper and lower segments; upper segment thickens and shortens, lower segment thins and elongates; in obstructed labour the exaggerated retraction ring is palpable above the symphysis pubis – a Bandl's ring

Rhesus factor (Rh) – 'Rhesus-positive' denotes the presence of an antigen on the red blood cells; present in 85% of the UK population; antibodies built up against this antigen by a Rhesus-negative woman can pass across the placenta and damage Rhesus-positive fetal red blood cells: this is called 'Rhesus incompatibility' (see **Anti-D immunoglobulin, Kleihauer test** and **Jaundice**)

Rotation – where the fetal head moves round through part of a circle to come under the free space of the pubic arch during the mechanism of labour

Runner, the – operating theatre helper (a health-care assistant, student) fetching essential supplies/equipment and dealing with odd jobs during surgical procedures

SANDS – Stillbirth and Neonatal Death Society

Save serum – venous blood is sent to the laboratory in a plain tube, i.e. without an anti-clotting agent. Once the blood is clotted, the serum is saved to enable blood to be cross-matched rapidly in an emergency, rather than completing the cross-matching when the blood may not be needed

SB – stillbirth – beware of possible confusion with next abbreviation (see **Serum bilirubin**)

SB/SBR – serum bilirubin, i.e. levels of bilirubin in blood – often written on a laboratory request form (Note also the earlier use of SB)

SC – subcutaneous – an injection under the skin

SCBU – special care baby unit – today used less than NNU/ NNICU

Schedule drugs – drugs in the five Controlled Drugs Schedules (Misuse of Drugs Regulations 2001), e.g. pethidine, morphine, diamorphine, barbiturates

Schultz method of placental separation – placenta lies in the upper part of the uterus – contraction/retraction reduces placental site, placenta partially separates, the weight causes descent to lower segment, membranes peel off behind it, fetal surface appears at vulva; uterine muscle contraction/retraction minimises blood loss (compare with Matthews Duncan separation)

Scriver test (see also **Guthrie test**) – PKU screening test; blood collected on the 8th or 9th or 10th day on to filter paper (see **Heel prick** in Section 2); overnight electrophoresis using chemicals allows separation of amino acids according to their molecular weight. Biochemical chromatography (colour) stains separate amino acids, enabling identification of deviations from normal, e.g. phenylketonuria and other inborn errors of metabolism

Scrub – specific hand/lower arm washing technique using antiseptic soap or gel solution, prior to putting on sterile gloves before aseptic/surgical procedures

SDS – surfactant deficiency syndrome (see subsequent entry)

Second-degree tear – perineal trauma involving the vaginal mucosa and skin and both superficial and deep muscles of the perineal body (see **Perineal/surrounding area trauma** in Section 2)

Sexually transmitted infection *(disease)* **(STI – STD)** – organisms spread by sexual contact (see Section 2 and **Infection – maternal, Infection – neonatal** and **Antenatal screening** in Section 2)

SFD – small for dates – the baby is SGA/light for dates (see **Intrauterine growth restriction (retardation)** in Section 2)

SGA – small for gestational age or SFD

SHO – senior house officer – a junior doctor with some medical experience; many are undertaking obstetric training before beginning work as a GP

Shock – generally a temporary state of massive physiological reaction to bodily damage/emotional trauma; characterised by a cold sweat, reduced blood pressure, rapid pulse and depression of vital processes, e.g. respiration; urgent action may be necessary to prevent compromise of mother and/or fetus

Shoulder presentation – transverse fetal lie, with shoulder lowermost in the uterus

SIDS – sudden infant death syndrome (see Section 2)

Sinciput – the brow, i.e. the area from the supra-orbital ridges to the coronal suture

Slow labour – a misleading lay term – the mother is not in established labour, i.e. the active phase of the first stage (see earlier entry), but is either in the latent phase or just having regular Braxton Hicks contractions (see earlier entry) that are painful

Spalding's sign – gross overlapping of fetal skull bones following death *in utero* (IUD) – manifestation usually takes 48 hours – seen on X-ray (see **Intrauterine death** in Section 2)

SPD – symphysis pubis diastasis – separation of the bones of the symphysis pubis joint (see **Symphysis pubis pain** in Section 2)

SRM or SROM – spontaneous rupture of membranes

Status eclampticus – repeated eclamptic convulsions without resting phase in between; life-threatening; may lead to fetal/maternal death (see **Eclampsia** in Section 2)

Status epilepticus – serious condition; repeated epileptic convulsions without resting phase in between; ? life threatening to the woman during pregnancy; considered less harmful to the fetus than eclamptic fits (see **Epilepsy** in Section 2)

Stillbirth – the complete expulsion of a baby >24 weeks which does not breathe, cry or show any other signs of life (see **Intrauterine death** and **Stillbirth and Neonatal Death Society** in Section 2)

Stillbirth rate – number of stillborn babies per 1000 total births (i.e. babies both alive and stillborn). Rate was 5.3 in the United Kingdom in 2006 (CEMACH 2008); 5.1 in England and Wales in 2008 (Office for National Statistics 2010)

Subinvolution – uterus does not involute at the expected rate following delivery; ? result of retained products of conception or blood clots; uterine infection; uterus, ? bulky, tender to touch, ? lochia offensive/remains rubra (see **Postnatal observations – mother** in Section 2)

Succenturiate lobe – a placenta with an extra cotyledon in the membranes with its own blood supply from the main placenta (see **Placental examination** in Section 2)

Supine hypotensive syndrome – compression of the inferior vena cava from the gravid uterus when the woman lies flat on her back; BP falls, woman feels faint, nauseated, is pale/clammy; – sitting her up/turning her on to left side relieves pressure/allows recovery

Surfactant/surfactant deficiency syndrome (SDS) – absence of the surface-acting agent allowing the alveoli to remain expanded when the first breath is taken, causing a syndrome (see **Respiratory distress syndrome** in Section 2)

Sutures of the fetal skull – incomplete ossification areas, leaving membranous spaces between the skull bones; where more than two suture lines meet – fontanelles

SPD – symphysis pubis diastasis – separation of the bones of the symphysis pubis (see **Symphysis pubis pain** in Section 2)

Syndrome – collection of signs and symptoms indicative of a disorder

Syntocinon (*synto*) – synthetic oxytocin; acts quickly on the uterus to produce contractions; used in IVI to induce/augment labour; may also be used intravenously in a single dose in PPH (see **Oxytocic drugs**, **Ergometrine** and **Syntometrine**)

Syntometrine – synthetic oxytocic agent containing 0.5 mg ergometrine and 5 IU (international units) syntocinon; given IM after the appearance of the anterior shoulder (i.e. active management of third stage); acts within 2 minutes, but produces a sustained uterine contraction (see **Oxytocic drugs**, **Ergometrine** and **Syntocinon**)

Tachycardia – increase in the heart rate; adult >100 beats per minute (e.g. in anaemia or after haemorrhage), fetal >160 beats per minute (see **Fetal distress** and **Cardiotocography**, baseline tachycardia in Section 2)

Tachypnoea – increase in the respiratory rate – adult >30 per minute, infant >60 per minute; neonatal transient tachypnoea – respiratory rate >60 per minute on a number of occasions without underlying pathology

TBA – traditional birth attendant – (see **Safe Motherhood Initiative** in Section 2)

TCI – 'to come in' – admit to hospital

TDS/tid – (*ter in die*) three times a day – often on a prescription

TED (thrombo-embolic disorder) stockings – thick elastic stockings (usually white) used to help maintain lower limb support to help prevent DVT

Term/full term – pregnancy that has reached 37 completed weeks of gestation

Termination of pregnancy (TOP) – the products of conception are expelled from the uterus by artificial means, i.e. surgically/medically with drugs

Third-degree tear – involves the vaginal mucosa, superficial and deep muscles of the perineal body and the anal sphincter (see **Perineal/surrounding area trauma** in Section 2)

TORCH – acronym for intrauterine infections; toxoplasmosis, others, rubella (a notifiable disease), cytomegalovirus, herpes (see **Infection – maternal**, **Infection – neonatal** and **Antenatal screening** in Section 2)

Toxaemia – a no-longer accepted term (see **Pre-eclampsia** and **Pregnancy-induced hypertension** in Section 2)

Trial of labour – when there is doubt about the ability of the fetal head to pass through the maternal pelvis during labour; effective uterine contractions, descent, flexion and some degree of moulding may enable head progression (see **CPD**)

Trial of scar – labour is allowed to start spontaneously (if possible) in a woman with a caesarean section scar to see if vaginal delivery is achievable; close monitoring of fetal and maternal conditions is essential

Trumpet – refers to the **Pinard** fetal stethoscope

TSA – **'to see again'** – often written in case notes

TTA, TTH, TTO – **'to take away/home/out'** (usually medication)

Tubes – usually refers to a stethoscope – occasionally Fallopian (uterine) tubes

Turner's syndrome – karyotype XO with female characteristics; ? presents with neck webbing, wide-angled elbows, protuberant abdomen, lower limb oedema, mental retardation; ? undiagnosed until failure to develop secondary sex characteristics/menstruation in teenage years

U & E – blood test for **urea and electrolytes** to ascertain renal function

US or USS – **ultrasound/ultrasound scan** – echoes of high-frequency sound waves form electronic images of body structures (see **Antenatal screening** in Section 2)

UTI – **urinary tract infection** (see Section 2)

Valsalva manoeuvre – the woman is asked to take a deep breath, hold it and push down with all her strength until she cannot push any longer; originally used as a method for expelling pus from the ears; was used as a form of directed pushing during second stage of labour until fairly recently

Vasa praevia – where the blood vessels from a succenturiate lobe run across the internal os of the cervix when the membranes are intact (velamentous insertion). If the membranes rupture, the blood vessels also rupture, causing fetal haemorrhage

VDRL – **Venereal Disease Research Laboratory** (see **Infection – maternal**, **Infection – neonatal** and **Antenatal screening** in Section 2)

VE – **vaginal examination**

Velamentous insertion – where the blood vessels from the cord run through the membranes before being inserted into the fetal surface of the placenta (see **Placental examination** in Section 2)

Venereal disease (VD) – terminology formerly used for sexually transmitted infections (diseases) (STIs), especially gonorrhoea/syphilis (see **Infection – maternal**, **Infection – neonatal** and **Antenatal screening** in Section 2)

Ventouse – a suction cap made of silicone plastic (silastic). It fits on to the baby's head rather like a skull cap. Once the cap has been positioned, the air is sucked out of it by means of a vacuum. Steady gentle traction during a contraction facilitates the delivery.

Vernix caseosa – white, lard-type substance covering the fetal skin *in utero* to protect against possible damage from being in a watery environment – some may still be present at birth

Version – correction of the fetal presentation; external cephalic version (ECV); the fetus is pushed head over heels externally (breech to head); offered to women at 36 weeks gestation (NICE 2008a); internal podalic version – vaginally during labour a transverse lie is converted to breech by pulling a leg down (see **Presentation** in this section and **Breech delivery** in Section 2)

Vertex – circular area on skull vault that presents when the head is well flexed, bounded by anterior and posterior fontanelles and parietal eminences on either side (see **Abdominal palpation** and **Delivery technique** in Section 2)

Viable/viability – capable of independent life, 24 weeks pregnancy in the United Kingdom

Vital statistics – statistics relating to life, death, disease; UK statistics include fertility rate, live births, stillbirths, perinatal, neonatal, post-neonatal and infant mortality rates and maternal mortality/morbidity

VKDB – **vitamin K deficiency bleeding** (see **Haemorrhagic disease** in Section 2)

Zygosity, determining – determining whether twins are identical (monozygous – derived from one single fertilised ovum) or fraternal (dizygous – derived from two different fertilised ova)

Zygote – the cell formed when the nuclear materials of the ovum and sperm unite

Section 2

Quick reference topics

This section of the book contains an alphabetical list of a wide variety of quick reference topics from basic midwifery and nursing procedures to obstetric and medical conditions, including emergency situations that may occur during the childbearing continuum. It also contains information on organisations that offer information for parents and professionals on specific conditions, e.g. Down's syndrome, and support services.

Abdominal palpation

Aim

- Assess uterine growth
- Determine fetal number, lie, presentation, position, attitude
- Assess presenting part engagement
- Locate/count fetal heart
- Reassure the mother

A Pocket Guide for Student Midwives: Second edition, by Stella McKay-Moffat and Pam Lee. © 2010 by John Wiley & Sons Ltd.

Preparation

- Inform woman of procedure; gain consent
- Ensure her bladder is empty
- Expose abdomen from xiphisternum to pubic hair line
- Wash hands/stand on the woman's right

Action

- Inspection – size, shape, scars, skin changes, FM
- Palpate fundal height – often measured with a tape from symphysis to fundus
- Chart fundal height (Gardosi and Francis 1999; NICE 2008a)
- Fundal palpation – ? head or breech in fundus
- Lateral palpation – locate a firm unbroken surface, the back
- Pelvic palpation – confirm presentation, assess engagement of presenting part
- Auscultation – Pinard's stethoscope – locate fetal heart over fetal back, below maternal umbilicus if head presentation, above if breech presentation; listen to rate, rhythm and volume for 1 minute
- Explain findings and encourage mother to feel her baby
- Document appropriately

Student activity

- Note the research about assessing fundal height
- Further reading: Gibson (2008)

Active management of labour

Function

- Prevent prolonged labour, maternal/fetal compromise
- Reduce instrumental/operative deliveries
- Improve woman's personal attention

Assessing/monitoring progress

- Labour onset – accurate labour diagnosis essential
- Present contractions – frequency, strength, length, regularity

- When/whether membranes ruptured
- Maternal condition:
  - (i) physical – well-being, pain, vital signs, fluid balance, urinalysis
  - (ii) psychological – coping ability, needs/wishes
- Fetal condition:
  - (i) FH/CTG (see guideline: NICE 2007)
  - (ii) presenting part position/descent
  - (iii) clear/meconium liquor
  - (iv) blood pH
- VE: progress noted on partograph

If progress of labour is slow, augmentation/acceleration of labour in uncomplicated cases may become part of a midwife's sphere of practice, depending on local protocols (see Rule 6 in NMC (2004)).

Student activity

Further reading: Sadler *et al.* (2001).

Administration of drugs

Aim

- Administer medication safely
- Keep accurate records
- Observe the effects of the medication

Preparation for all methods

- Collect prescription sheet
- Check drug administration record to ensure medication is not already given
- Check each prescribed drug for:
  - (i) date prescribed
  - (ii) drug name, form, dose, expiry date
  - (iii) route of administration
  - (iv) specific directions for use
  - (v) time(s) due
  - (vi) client drug sensitivity
  - (vii) doctor's signature

- Adhere to hospital policy for:
  (i) injection site
  (ii) administration of controlled drugs
  (iii) who can give IV injections (students do not normally give IV or IVI drugs)

Action

Oral

- Identify woman/seek consent
- Once drug checked by trained staff, place selected drug in container
- Give to woman to take, with a drink prn
- Ensure drug is swallowed
- Record drug administration/response on appropriate chart

IM/SC injection

- Identify woman/seek consent
- Ensure appropriate drug/dosage – check by trained staff
- Prepare needle and syringe for injection
- Draw up drug aseptically/place needle and syringe in receiver
- Swab skin prn
- Insert needle and withdraw plunger to ensure no blood is drawn
- Administer drug
- Observe for effect
- Record appropriately

Controlled drug

- Two qualified staff members to check ampoule/tablets
- Count stock remaining – record in controlled drugs book
- At woman's bedside check ID labels/seek consent
- Drug administered as previously
- Record drug given in case notes/on prescription sheet
- Record as drug given and witnessed in the controlled drugs book
- Observe/record effects of medication

Intravenous injections

- Check drug details/dilution/infusion
- Check fluid/equipment
- Two staff members identify client/seek consent
- Ensure appropriate drug/dosage
- Draw up aseptically
- Administer at prescribed rate, usually through cannula port; sometimes directly IV
- Observe/record effects of medication (NB: onset likely to be rapid)
- Record drug given in case notes/on prescription sheet

Adding to infusion bag

As for IV injection but:

(i) stop infusion

(ii) add to bag and shake

(iii) label correctly

(iv) check infusion rate for administration

(v) recommence at given rate

Giving via a syringe driver

As for IV injection but:

(i) make volume up with suitable dilution prn

(ii) prime infusion tube before measuring the barrel length of medication to be infused

(iii) set rate according to prescribed dose/maker's instructions

(iv) set/check rate with prescription sheet – start the pump

(v) check pump, cannula, tubing at least 4 hourly

Student activity

- Ensure you have a copy of *Standards for Medicine Management* (NMC 2007), *Record Keeping: Guidance for Nurses and Midwives* (NMC 2009), *Midwives' Rules and Standards* (NMC 2004)

- Note your unit policy on drug administration and standing orders
- Further reading: Dimond (2006) Chapter 20

Admission in labour

Aim

- Ascertain physical condition
- Determine whether labour is established
- Alleviate fear/anxiety
- Facilitate care planning
- Offer support prn

Preparation

- Ensure privacy
- Read woman's hand-held notes/case record
- Ensure that maternal/fetal monitoring equipment is available

Action

- Follow recorded special instructions
- Perform quick assessment – is delivery imminent?
  (1) yes – take straight to delivery room and proceed
  (2) no – explain/complete admission procedure
    (i) take history of onset of labour
    (ii) perform 'top to toe' examination
    (iii) ask whether bowels open/test urine sample
    (iv) palpate abdomen
    (v) assess contraction frequency, strength, duration, mother's response
    (vi) VE prn with woman's consent
    (vii) inform woman and partner of findings
    (viii) discuss plans for rest of care
    (ix) keep accurate records
    (x) fetal heart monitoring ? routine admission procedure

Student activity

Note your unit's policy for admission; observe records for documenting admission in labour.

Adoption

Legislation

- First Adoption Act 1926
- Subsequent Acts 1958; 1968; 1976
- Children Act 1975 (Part I); 1989
- Adoption and Children Act 2002
- The Children and Adoption Act 2006 (England and Wales)

See the Acts on the Office of Public Sector Information website on http://www.opsi.gov.uk/

Welfare principle

The child's long- and short-term welfare and, wherever possible, its feelings should be taken into consideration.

Role of local authority

- Has the power to make and participate in arrangements for the adoption and placing of children who are not in care for adoption
- Supervises children intended for adoption
- Appoints a Guardian *ad litem* as child's advocate, usually an experienced social worker, in a contested adoption or if there are High Court proceedings, and as a court adviser
- Provides counselling service for adoptees wishing to apply for their original birth certificate

Who can adopt?

- Married couples (including same-sex), one of whom must be over 21 and the other over 18 years, unless they are the mother or father of the child
- Must be resident in the United Kingdom
- Single person over 21 years of age (there must be special grounds for a man to adopt a female child unless he is the partner of the child's mother)
- One partner of a pair if the spouse cannot be found or has mental illness

• Same-sex partners are able to adopt since the Civil Partnership Act 2004. (See the Act on the Office of Public Sector Information website on http://www.opsi.gov.uk/)

Children for adoption

• Must be free for adoption, under 18 and not married
• Parental consent must be given unless:
  (i) parent dead or missing
  (ii) parent withholding consent unreasonably
  (iii) parent guilty of persistently or seriously ill-treating child
  (iv) child living with adoptive parents for 5 years
  (v) natural father of child

Procedure for adoption

• Parents – both natural and adoptive – *must* understand that it is legal, binding and permanent
• The new Act provides for support services for these parents

Placement of child

• With local authority adoption service
• With voluntary adoption agency (approved)
• Direct placement only if relative of child

Process

• *Natural mother* contacts Social Services Department or hospital social worker (in pregnancy) regarding adoption – formal consent obtained after baby reaches 6 weeks
• *Doctor* certifies mother's general and mental health and provides details of pregnancy, labour and other relevant factors
• *Prospective adoptive parents* apply to adoption agency
• *Adoption agency* investigates prospective parents' suitability; tries to 'match' babies to parents; advises and helps both natural and adoptive parents with legal aspects; respects natural parents' wishes regarding religious upbringing

- *Local authority* must be notified of intention to adopt at least 13 weeks before adoption order can be made, to enable investigations
- *Baby for adoption*
  - physically examined, any defects noted, adoptive parents informed
  - placed with foster parents or may remain with mother (often in mother and baby unit)
  - placed with adoptive parents when *6 weeks* old or possibly on discharge from hospital, but no consent can be given before 6 weeks in case mother changes her mind
  - lives with adoptive parents for *13 weeks*, enabling investigations and home visits and thus ensuring suitability
  - *The Court* (High Court, County Court, Children and Family Court)
  - Ensures:
    (i) that mother consents to the adoption
    (ii) that adoption is in the best interest of the child
    (iii) that no reward was given to the mother by the adoptive parents
  - Appoints the Children and Family Court Advisory and Support Person for the purposes of any relevant application – the officer appointed:
    (i) acts on behalf of the child and safeguards its interests
    (ii) prepares a child welfare report
    (iii) witnesses documents
    (iv) performs prescribed functions
  - Grants, refuses or postpones for 2 years the adoption order, depending on circumstances

Other points

- Natural parent needs a court order to remove child living with adoptive parents or foster parents prior to adoption
- If an adoption agency is not involved, i.e. if the child is placed by the High Court or if it is a foster child and consent has been given – child must have lived with adoptive parents for *12 months* as part of the family and must have been visited in the home
- If no parental consent is given, child must have lived with adoptive parents for *5 years*

- If a child is being adopted from another country, then the laws of that country must be followed
- Adoption proceedings will be heard in private
- When 18, the adoptee can apply to the Registrar's Office for information necessary for obtaining his/her original birth certificate
- If a child is placed with an adoption agency but is not adopted after 1 year, the natural parents can apply to resume control, but the Court has to be satisfied that the child will be looked after properly. If the parent does not want to resume control – then the LA looks after the child
- The 2002 Act emphasises avoiding delay, and the agencies involved in the adoption have to:
  - (i) draw up a timetable of events
  - (ii) provide directions to ensure the timetable is adhered to
- The Act 'tightens up' loopholes so that children do not get lost in the system and are not moved from one carer to another unnecessarily
- The Children and Adoption Act 2006 introduces a number of provisions with regard to arranging contact with children following parental separation and with regard to adoption with a foreign element
- Parents may be entitled to Statutory Adoption Leave and Statutory Adoption Pay similar to maternity pay and leave (see **Maternity benefits**)

Amniocentesis

Not a midwife's procedure.

Aim

- Aseptic removal of liquor sample for investigation
- Reassure mother/allay fears
- Prevent Rhesus incompatibility

Preparation

- Explain procedure to woman/partner
- Obtain consent

- Ultrasound room ready
- Ensure client privacy/safety
- Trolley prepared:
    (i) correct pack
    (ii) needles and syringes
    (iii) sample bottles
    (iv) local anaesthetic
    (v) dressings/plastic spray
    (vi) cleansing solution

Management

Observations of mother/fetus prior to procedure.

Action

- Assist doctor with equipment preparation
- Reassure mother, act as advocate prn
- Assist doctor with procedure prn
- Observe mother/fetus following procedure
- Keep accurate records
- Give IM anti-D immunoglobulin 250 IU if Rhesus negative/status unknown
- Escort to ward/couch for rest/observation
- Inform woman of signs/symptoms of miscarriage and action to take if present

Student activity

List indications for performing amniocentesis.

Amniotic Fluid Embolus (AFE)

Aetiology

AFE occurs when amniotic fluid is forced into maternal circulation via the uterine sinuses of the placental bed. Most likely to occur during delivery.

Diagnosis

• Difficult to diagnose clinically; usually confirmed on postmortem when fetal squames and lanugo are found in maternal lungs
• Early symptoms:
   (i) dyspnoea
   (ii) restlessness
   (iii) panic
   (iv) feeling cold
   (v) paraesthesia ('pins and needles')
• Collapse likely
• Placental abruption may occur, resulting in fetal death (compare with pulmonary embolus – see Viles (2007); **embolism**)

Risk factors

• Older women
• Multiparous
• Strong contractions of uterus
• Oxytocic drugs – augmentation or induction
• Multiple pregnancy
• Polyhydramnios
• Rare cases following amniocentesis

Sequelae

• DIC is a real problem; AF contains high levels of thromboplastin; if woman survives initial embolism, may die from coagulation failure; amniotic fluid depresses uterine activity and hypotonic uterus may lead to bleeding
• Death – CEMACH (Lewis 2007) report noted an inexplicable rise in deaths from AFE: 17 women died in 2003–2005; previously only 5 deaths in 2000–2002 (Lewis 2004)

Management

• Medical aid
• Commence CPR if necessary

- Administer oxygen
- Set up IVI
- CVP line inserted
- Transfer to ICU if possible
- Mechanical ventilation
- Caesarean section even if fetus dead – easier to resuscitate woman if uterus empty
- Support partner/family

Prevention

- Difficult – said to be a rare and largely unavoidable condition
- Careful use of oxytocic drugs
- Induction and augmentation of labour kept to minimum

Student activity

Further reading: Viles (2007).

Anaemia

A deficiency in the quality or quantity of the red blood cells (RBCs) (erythrocytes), and therefore in the oxygen-carrying capacity of the blood. Hb (haemoglobin) of 11 g (grams per decilitre, i.e. per 100 ml) at booking/during the first trimester or $10.5 \text{ g} \geq 28$ weeks indicates anaemia and needs further investigation (NICE 2008a).

Aetiology

- Iron deficiency – poor diet, malabsorption
- Folic acid deficiency
- B12 deficiency (pernicious anaemia)
- Haemoglobinopathies, i.e. abnormal haemoglobin, e.g. sickle cell anaemia
- Blood loss – acute, i.e. haemorrhage, or chronic, e.g. due to infection
- Aplastic anaemia – inability to produce rbc
- Blood disorders, e.g. leukaemia

Signs and symptoms

- Possibly asymptomatic, i.e. no obvious symptoms
- Tiredness, lethargy
- Pallor, i.e. of skin and inside of lower eyelid
- Breathlessness
- Fainting
- Tachycardia
- Frequent infections

Investigations

- History
- Blood film (FBC) – Hb, serum folate, serum ferritin, red cell picture (size, colour, maturity – see **MCH** and **MCV** in Section 1)

Management

- Depends on cause and blood picture
- Correct known cause
- Iron prn (historically iron was given *routinely* in pregnancy)
- Folic acid – all women should take 400 µg (mcg) daily before conception and for first 12 weeks gestation (NICE 2008b)

Possible complications

- Poor general health and resistance to infection
- Inability to withstand haemorrhage
- Perinatal and maternal mortality/morbidity

Student activity

Further reading: NICE (2008a, 2008b); Ursell (2005).

Antenatal screening

- Screening is the examination of an asymptomatic population to detect the development of a condition in those in whom the disease is already present

• There should be set criteria to determine who should be screened for what
• Tests should be safe, simple, quick and cheap, providing repeatable, valid results
• Antenatal screening is *offered* to all pregnant women, but may lead to anxiety as well as reassurance

Routine tests and examinations

Abdominal examination

• To determine symphysis–fundal distance to estimate fetal size and growth from 24 weeks gestation (NICE 2008a)
• Auscultation of fetal heart routinely not recommended (NICE 2008a) but may be done at mother's request

Blood pressure measurement

Usually at every visit.

Weight and height

To calculate body mass index (BMI) at booking (NICE 2008a) – see Section 1 for calculation.

Urinalysis

• At every visit for protein and glucose
• MSSU at booking for asymptomatic bacteruria (NICE 2008a)

Blood tests

• ABO and Rhesus group (if Rhesus negative, the partner may be offered screening)
• Rhesus antibodies at booking and at 28 weeks
• Haemoglobin at booking and at 28 weeks (see **Anaemia**)
• Haemoglobinopathies (see website under *Student activity* below)
• Rubella titre (to assess immunity) at booking
• VDRL – for syphilis

- hCG, AFP, uE3, inhibin-A (part of Down's syndrome screening – see NICE (2008a))
- Hepatitis B (a notifiable disease), hepatitis C
- HIV

Ultrasound scan

- Ideally 10–13 weeks (NICE 2008a) for gestation and nuchal translucency (part of Down's syndrome screening)
- At 18–20 weeks for anomalies

Additional tests offered when necessary

- Amniocentesis (see earlier text)
- Biophysical profile (see **Fetal distress**)
- Blood sugar (see **Diabetes**)
- Chorionic villus sampling (see subsequent section)
- Haemoglobinopathies (see subsequent section)
- Vaginal swab for infection, e.g. *Candida*, *Chlamydia*, gonorrhoea
- Toxoplasmosis (see **Infection – neonatal**)

Student activity

- Further reading: NICE (2008a); Sickle Cell Society on http://www.sicklecellsociety.org
- Sickle cell and thalassaemia screening programme on http://sct.screening.nhs.uk

Antepartum haemorrhage

Causes

Lower genital tract

- Infection
- Trauma (accident or assault)
- Cervical abnormalities, e.g. ectopy (erosion), polyp (small fleshy growth), CIN (see Section 1)

Upper genital tract

- Placental abruption (placenta separating)
- Placenta praevia (placenta in the lower uterine segment)
- Trauma, e.g. road accident
- Uterine rupture
- Ruptured vasa praevia (placental vessel in amniotic sac below presenting part)

Predisposing or risk factors

- History of miscarriage, abortion or caesarean section
- High parity and older age
- Cocaine use and smoking
- Hypertensive disorders
- Multiple pregnancy
- Domestic violence

Management

See Figure 1.
- Depends on:
    (i) diagnosis
    (ii) severity of bleeding
    (iii) fetal/maternal conditions
- Not midwife-led care – medical aid in accordance with a midwife's responsibility and sphere of practice (Rule 6 in *Midwives' Rules and Standards*: NMC 2004)

Complications

- Risk of uterine infection
- Shock, compromising mother and baby
- DIC
- Perinatal death
- Maternal death
- Psychological morbidity, e.g. post-traumatic stress

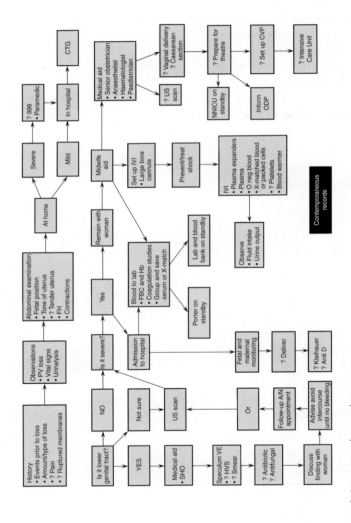

Figure 1 Antepartum haemorrhage.

Student activity

- Note your local policies and procedures for APH
- Further reading: Boyle (2002); Liston (2007)

Arterial blood pressure recording

Aim

Measure/record/monitor arterial blood pressure.

Preparation

- Explain procedure to client/gain consent
- Check previous recordings
- Check whether sphygmomanometer (sphyg.)/BP recording device is working
- Client in suitable position
- Ensure correct size cuff

Action

- Expose arm/palpate antecubital fossa for pulse
- Position sphyg. at approximately heart height
- Secure cuff around upper arm (ensuring large enough) and inflate – note when radial pulse obliterated and inflate to 20 mmHg above this level

Release valve

(i) systolic BP – first sound
(ii) diastolic BP – when sound changes, i.e. Korotkoff 4 (K4) or when sound disappears, i.e. Korotkoff 5 (K5)
(NB: K4 is commonly used in pregnancy for greater accuracy (conflicting views); K5 is recorded by automated sphyg.)

- Electric sphyg. – ensure microphone placed over brachial artery/follow instructions
- Disconnect equipment
- Leave client comfortable
- Record findings accurately/inform client

Student activity

- Revise normal BP mechanism control/physiological changes during pregnancy
- Further reading: Higgins and de Swiet (2001)

Artificial feeds – bottle feeding

Aim

- To ensure formula feeds are reconstituted correctly
- To reduce the risk of infection due to poor hygiene
- To ensure adequate infant nutrition

Preparation

- Prepare clean working surface
- Explain procedure to mother
- Ensure equipment sterilised
- Boil water – allow to cool to a maximum of hand-hot
- Wash hands

Action

- Remove bottles/teats from steriliser, ensuring no contamination
- Read instructions on the sides of formula packet – determine quantity of feed required
- Put correct amount of *cooled* boiled water into bottle
- Using scoop provided, fill with powder and level off with knife
- Put scoop of powder into bottle, repeat prn
- Put cap and teat on, shake vigorously
- Allow to cool, test temperature on inside of wrist before giving
- If several bottles being made up, put teats inside bottle
- Once at room temperature, store in 'fridge' until required
- Ensure mother understands baby should be held during feed and not 'propped up' in a pushchair/cot

Student activity

• Familiarise yourself with reports on infant feeding and **Baby Friendly Initiative**
• Further reading: Renfrew *et al.* (2008)

Artificial rupture of membranes (ARM)

Forewater amniotomy; also see **Augmentation/acceleration of labour** in Section 1 and **Induction of labour**.

Aim

• To rupture forewaters in order to accelerate labour
• To exclude abnormalities, e.g. meconium liquor

Preparation

• Ensure privacy/maintain dignity
• Explain procedure/seek consent (Dimond 2006; NMC 2008)
• Trolley prepared
• Dressing pack
• Sterile cleansing solution
• Device for rupturing membranes (Amnihook/amnicot)
• Sterile pads
• Pinard's stethoscope/Sonicaid
• Abdominal palpation
• Comfortable position

Action

• Woman's bladder should be empty, vulva exposed
• Aseptic technique
• Swab vulva
• Vaginal examination – confirm:
  (i) dilatation of cervix
  (ii) presenting part

    (iii) no cord present

    (iv) forewaters intact

- With two fingers of right hand in vagina:
  - (i) guide device to forewaters, avoiding vaginal trauma
  - (ii) wait for contraction and bulging forewaters (if possible)
  - (iii) rupture membranes
  - (iv) remove device, avoiding trauma
  - (v) fetal scalp electrode (FSE) applied prn
  - (vi) check liquor draining/clear
  - (vii) exclude cord prolapse
  - (viii) remove fingers/place clean pad over vulva
- Listen to fetal heart
- Advise mother of findings and make her comfortable
- Record procedure accurately, including indications for ARM (NMC 2009)

Student activity

Further reading: NICE (2007); NMC (2004, 2007, 2008, 2009)

Aseptic technique

Aim

Reduce contamination risk during procedures

Preparation

- Inform client of procedure/gain consent (NMC 2008)
- Clean dressing trolley – from top downwards
- Sterile solution/other necessary equipment on lower shelf
- Place sterile pack on top of trolley – check expiry date
- Open carefully, secure outer bag to trolley for disposal of swabs
- Ensure privacy/maintain client dignity

Action

- Wash hands
- Open inner pack carefully/prepare equipment prn

- Maintain clean field/area of appropriate body part
- Wash hands again or use surgical rub
- Use sterile gloves/forceps for procedure
- Dispose of soiled swabs/forceps safely
- Document actions/observations
- Ensure client is comfortable following procedure

Augmentation/acceleration of labour

Also see **Induction of labour – alternative and 'natural'** and **Induction of labour – medical**.

- Medically enhancing spontaneous labour when progress is slow/failed
- ARM (see earlier text) and IV cannulation may be part of the midwife's sphere of practice (see Rule 6: NMC (2004), *Midwives' Rules and Standards*)
- First identify cause (see **Prolonged labour – first stage**)

Methods

ARM (forewater amniotomy)

Once performed delivery is committed.
- *Indications*:
  - woman's informed consent
  - labour established
  - cervix ≥ 4 cm dilated
  - slow progress
  - inadequate contractions
  - for liquor examination
  - application of FSE
- *Contraindications*
  - if woman objects
  - cervix < 4 cm dilated
  - spurious labour – i.e. not established
  - high presenting part
  - complications

- *Advantages of ARM*
  - ? shortens labour (no consensus in research)
  - liquor observation
  - FSE application
  - Absence of bulging forewaters may enable closer application of the cervix to the head
  - may increase dilatation and stimulate prostaglandin release
- *Disadvantages of ARM*
  - stress and anxiety during procedure
  - cervical/vaginal wall trauma
  - fetal hypoxia from cord compression/prolapse
  - fetal bradycardia due to fall in placental perfusion/head compression
  - maternal shock if sudden large drainage
  - discomfort from draining liquor
  - caput/cephalhaematoma formation
  - excess moulding
  - increased frequency/strength of contractions
  - increased pain/less able to cope/more analgesia
  - increased risk of intrauterine infection – maternal/neonatal infection
  - woman may feel a lack of control/decreased satisfaction
  - increased risk of amniotic fluid embolus
- *Possible advantages of intact membranes*
  - labour not committed
  - even pressure on fetus during contractions
  - less risk of infection
  - ? pain more tolerable

Syntocinon added to IVI

- With woman's informed consent (NMC 2008)
- Administered via an infusion pump for dose accuracy
- Before ARM or following ARM
- Initial slow rate gradually increases – stimulates uterine contractions to accelerate labour

Advantages

- shortens labour
- gives some control over labour
- readily stopped if complications arise
- increases chances of spontaneous vaginal delivery

Disadvantages

- increased frequency/strength of contractions
- increased pain/less able to cope/more analgesia
- lessens mobility/alternative positions
- continuous electronic fetal monitoring often applied
- over-stimulation/tonic contractions
- fluid overload (oxytocin has antidiuretic properties)
- ? increases neonatal jaundice
- increased risk of amniotic fluid embolus

Management

- Close monitoring of fetal/maternal well-being
- ? Continuous electronic fetal monitoring (see **CTG** in Section 1) (NICE 2007)
- Maternal vital signs
- Fluid balance
- Urinalysis for ketones
- IVI gradually increased until contractions are a maximum of 1 every 3–4 minutes; IVI ? decreased as labour progresses
- Ensure uterus relaxes between contractions
- Close monitoring of progress – contractions, abdominal examination, VE
- Usual care in labour
- ? Oral ranitidine (see **Mendelson's syndrome**)
- ? Only clear fluids orally
- Information/support for woman/partner
- Continue Syntocinon infusion for 1 hour after delivery (<PPH)

Student activity

- Note your local policy and procedures
- Familiarise yourself with labour records
- Revise physiology of labour
- Further reading: Sadler *et al.* (2001)

Basic life support (BLS) – adult

Actions taken in an emergency situation when the individual has respiratory or cardiac arrest.

NB: the following information is a *very simple guide* to adult BLS to act as a prompt to further reading/quick reminder of existing knowledge.

- Ensure victim, self and others are safe
- Check for response
- Shout for help/dial 999
- Thirty chest compressions initially
- Two rescue breaths via mouth to mouth or mouth to nose
- Continue ratio of 30 compressions (at rate of 100 per minute) to 2 breaths (Handley 2005)

BLS – in pregnancy

- A special situation requiring modification of process
- Chest compressions may be difficult in late pregnancy
- Avoid vascular compromise from gravid uterus, e.g. supine hypotension – tilt slightly to left lateral
- Early advanced airway maintenance needed, i.e. via endotracheal tube
- Rapid assistance from obstetrician and anaesthetist

Student activity

- Priority to read and clearly understand the procedure/situation; BLS may be required in pregnant and non-pregnant persons
- A life-saving essential skill; ensure you have frequent/regular simulated practice

• Familiarise yourself with the equipment in your hospital unit and community settings

• Further reading: Handley (2005); The Resuscitation Council (UK) website http://www.resus.org.uk

Birth asphyxia

See **Fetal distress** in Section 2 and **Apgar score** in Section 1.

• Failure to establish spontaneous breathing – with/without heartbeat

• The Apgar score is commonly used to determine severity of neonatal compromise (see Figure 2)

Aetiology

• Obstructed airway – liquor, mucus, blood, meconium
• Respiratory depression, e.g. due to pethidine, morphine, or GA
• Cerebral haemorrhage
• Congenital abnormalities, e.g. heart, lungs
• Prematurity – lack of surfactant in lungs (RDS/SDS); immature respiratory centre/system
• Severe intrauterine infection
• Pneumothorax (air in chest) or reflex apnoea due to mismanaged initial resuscitation

Management

Neonatal resuscitation; see Figure 3.

Sign	0	1	2	Score
Colour (appearance)	Pale/blue	Pink with blue extremities	Completely pink	
Apex beat (pulse)	Absent	Slow–less than 100	More than 100	
Response to stimuli (grimace)	No response	Facial grimace	Crying	
Muscle activity	Limp	Some flexion of limbs	Active movements	
Respiratory effort	Absent	Slow irregular cry	Strong cry	
			Total score	

Figure 2 Apgar score.

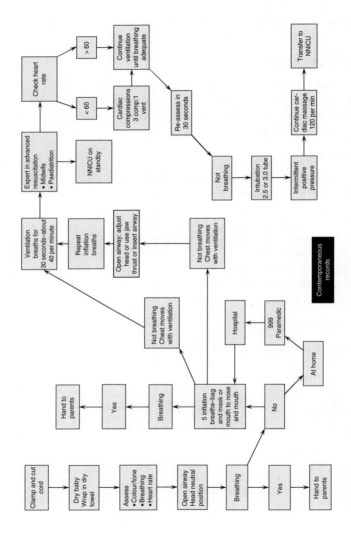

Figure 3 Neonatal resuscitation.

Bladder care in labour

Aim

- Prevent bladder damage during labour
- Prevent full bladder delaying progress
- Detect abnormalities in urine, e.g. ketones

Preparation

- Ensure privacy/maintain dignity
- Collect equipment prn – e.g. bed pans, urinalysis sticks
- Inform woman about emptying bladder at regular intervals

Action

- Early labour – encourage mobilisation and fluids prn
- Empty bladder 2–4 hourly, perform and record urinalysis
- If not mobile – offer bedpans at regular intervals 2–4 hourly
- If full bladder palpated/unable to empty – catheterise
- Prior to caesarean section – ? insert an indwelling catheter
- Prior to instrumental delivery – ? catheterisation (non-retaining)

Student activity

- Describe why a full bladder may cause problems in labour
- How may damage to the bladder be minimised?

Blood glucose monitoring (neonatal)

See **Heel prick**.

Blood pressure measuring

See **Arterial blood pressure recording**.

Bowel care in labour

Aim

- Prevent full rectum delaying labour progress
- Maintain dignity during the second stage of labour

Preparation

- During admission ask if her bowels opened prior to labour onset
- Explain importance of empty bowel in labour
- Seek consent if action is necessary

Action

- Collect receiver for equipment
  - (i) suppository/enemette
  - (ii) gloves, lubricating gel/warm water, gauze swabs
  - (iii) bedpan and cover (unless toilet is very close)
  - (iv) bedding protection
- Ensure privacy
- Woman in left lateral position, knees bent, buttocks exposed
- Protect bedding

Suppository

- Lubricate (lubricant on gauze)
- Locate anus, insert suppository 4.5 cm into the rectum using gloved index finger
- Instruct woman to hold suppository for as long as possible

Enemette

- Read instructions; snip off the top with clean scissors
- Lubricate end (lubricant on gauze); insert into anus
- Squeeze the contents into the rectum
- Cover the woman and leave as comfortable as possible
- Ensure call bell within easy reach
- Record administration, monitor effectiveness/results

NB: If labour is well established, perform VE prior to procedure.

Breast expression of milk

NB: not part of normal lactation management; may be performed if:
(i) baby is separated from the mother in NNU
(ii) baby is unable to 'fix' correctly at the breast
(iii) mother wishes to learn technique prior to return to work while maintaining breastfeeding
(iv) temporary medical indication, e.g. drug therapy
(v) temporary relief of milk engorgement (see **Breastfeeding**)

Aim

• Remove milk from the breast as comfortably as possible
• Prevent breast engorgement

Preparation

• Explain procedure to mother/seek consent (NMC 2008)
• Equipment sterilised; electric/hand pump, cups, tubing, container for milk
• Wash nipples prn
• Maintain privacy

Action

Mechanical/electric pump

• Place cup over nipple and areola
• Apply suction; check whether it is not too uncomfortable
• Check that the milk is being ejected into the correct place
• When breast fully expressed, stop suction, remove cup carefully, repeat on other breast

Manual expression

• Carried out by midwife/mother if no pump is available/woman prefers
• Seat woman comfortably – bed table/similar underneath breast
• Place sterile receiver beneath breast to catch milk

- Working from the periphery, both hands either side of the breast, massage with firm strokes towards the nipple
- Compress the areola and eject the milk into the receiver
- As one breast releases milk, the other may also leak – receiver/breast pad in place
- If the milk is being saved:
    - (i) place in a sterile bottle
    - (ii) cover
    - (iii) label
    - (iv) refrigerate/freeze

Student activity

- Note your local policies
- Further reading: Labiner-Wolf *et al.* (2008); Sweet (2008)

Breastfeeding

Aids to successful breastfeeding

Atmosphere

- Relaxed, unhurried, private, no interruptions
- Rest, family and professional support

Frequency

- Ideally within 1 hour of delivery
- Varies with baby – 1–8 hours, average is 3–4 hours
- Time suckling is according to milk amount/flow, baby's appetite
- Foremilk (early flow) – higher water and lower fat than more satisfying hindmilk

Position – mother

- Comfortable, relaxed (essential)
- Upright, supported by pillows (aids relaxation)

• Support arm holding baby (pillows on lap, on raised thigh – foot stool useful)
• Lateral position if there are perineal or abdominal wounds

Position – baby

Head on upper arm, body across mother's chest or vertically, with baby's nearest arm tucked round mother's chest under her arm or 'back to front', i.e. body under arm, buttocks on a pillow with arm across chest, baby's head positioned for clear nostrils.

Breast

• ? Supported and/or lifted from below
• Point nipple at roof of baby's mouth; if no rooting reflex, stroke the baby's lips with nipple, or cheek with finger
• Nipple and areola, especially underside, need to be grasped and drawn into baby's mouth
• ? Support heavy breast with cupped hand (prevents loss of fixing)
• If incorrectly fixed may cause pain; release vacuum using little finger in corner of mouth and press baby's jaw
• If correctly fixed, generally no discomfort to mother and small cheek muscle movement seen in front of baby's ear
• Ensure correct fixing after baby pauses

Diet

• No set restrictions
• Anecdotal evidence suggests that certain foods may give baby wind/colic/loose stools:
    (i) very spicy foods
    (ii) highly acidic foods, e.g. pickles and citric fruits/juices
    (iii) large quantities of chocolate
    (iv) some fruit and vegetables
• Effects seem to appear 6–48 hours after maternal consumption

• Alcohol levels in milk = maternal plasma alcohol levels; therefore minimal intake advised
• Tobacco chemicals and metabolites present in milk if mother actively/passively smokes

Drugs

The mother should inform her doctor or pharmacist before taking any medication.

The following list is not exhaustive, but includes drugs that are in common use:

• *Contraindications*
  ○ Aspirin
  ○ Oestrogen, e.g. combined oral contraceptive
  ○ Tetracycline
  ○ Vitamins D and A in high doses
  ○ Anticancer drugs
• *Caution*
  ○ Antidepressants (high doses)
  ○ Antihistamines
  ○ Co-trimoxazole (Septrin) antibiotics
  ○ Antimalarials
  ○ Corticosteroids (high doses)
  ○ Phenobarbitone
  ○ Anti-epilepsy drugs
• *Safe*
  ○ Antacids and bulk laxatives
  ○ Antibiotics – cephalosporins (Ceporex), erythromycin, nystatin, penicillins
  ○ Anticoagulants – heparin, warfarin
  ○ Ergometrine
  ○ Insulin
  ○ Metformin
  ○ Metronidazole (Flagyl) – normal doses
  ○ Paracetamol

- Progesterone – only contraceptives
- Vitamins B and C, folic acid
- Vitamins A and D (normal doses)

Complications

Information, encouragement and practical tips aid the overcoming of difficulties/continuation of breastfeeding.

Nipples

(1) Non-protractile (flat) or inverted – likely to make fixing difficult

Solutions

(1) Manual or electronic breast pump may draw nipple out to enable baby to fix

Soft nipple shield (sterilised), but this may reduce stimulation/ milk transfer

Express milk using pump (see above) and cup/spoon feed

(2) Sore/cracked, commonly owing to incorrect fixing (NB: if nipple bleeding, baby may vomit blood (mother's) following a feed – caution thrush (*Candida*) may develop in nipple increasing pain

(2) Rest nipple – express milk and cup feed

Change mother's/baby's position – correct fixing, soft nipple shield as above – anecdotal evidence suggests nipple cream may be soothing; antifungal cream if *Candida* suspected; breastfeeding on one side only

Engorgement

(1) Temporary vascular

Engorgement due to increased blood supply in days 2–4; breasts feel uniformly tender/painful, enlarged and possibly hot; ? slight transient pyrexia

Solutions

(1) Warm bathing in shower/ bath; hot and cold compresses; well-supporting bra; mild analgesics, e.g. paracetamol; dark green cabbage leaves in bra lessen swelling

(2) Milk engorgement
Due to blockage/failure of emptying – ? incorrect positioning. ? greater supply than demand – breasts may be generally/locally hard, tender/painful, hot/inflamed; blocked ampulla will feel like hard, pea-sized swelling causing tenderness behind areola (NB: be aware of mastitis–pyrexia; generally unwell, local pain, heat, medical aid and antibiotics)

(2) Correct fixing and/or change baby's position; hand express some milk to soften breasts enabling easier fixing; warm bathing, gentle massage with flat of hand all round breast to nipple before/between feeds; hand express but avoid over-stimulation; homeopathic remedies for inflammation – (Tiran & Mack 2000)
Continue feeding if no pus

Insufficient milk
Considered if baby is continually unable to settle and wanting feeding (not just now and again) and has a low urine output (disposable nappies may make observation of output difficult). Possibly due to inadequate breast development during pregnancy because of poor pituitary or placental hormone levels

Cause
(1) Poor lactation

Solution
(1) Correct fixing and frequent feeding aids stimulation; nutritious diet and adequate fluids

(2) Ineffective draught (let down) reflex due to inefficient neurohormonal regulation from:
(i) inadequate nipple stimulation due to poor fixing

(i) Correct fixing
Avoid complementary/supplementary feeding if possible – water or formula only if really necessary using cup/spoon feeding

(ii) psychological factors inhibiting hormone release e.g. tiredness, stress, anxiety, family pressure not to breastfeed

(ii) Plenty of rest and relaxation aided by supportive family; aromatherapy may be useful (Tiran & Mack 2000) or homeopathic remedies (Ayers 2000)

Breastfeeding Initiative (BFI)

Set up in 1991 by WHO and UNICEF (United Nations Children's Fund) promoting breastfeeding internationally. The initiative recommends Ten Steps to Successful Breastfeeding, while discouraging adverse practices. The Baby Friendly Hospital Initiative implements this policy, with 'Baby Friendly Hospital' status awarded if external assessors agree that the ten steps have been successfully completed. There is also a separate award for educational institutions.

Breech

Types

- Complete (flexed) – fetal knees and hips flexed, feet close to buttocks
- Extended (frank) – knees extended, feet by head
- Footling – one/both feet below buttocks (more common preterm)
- Knee presentation – one/both knees below buttocks (uncommon)

Positions

- Left/right sacro-anterior (LSA/RSA)
- Left/right sacro-posterior (LSP/RSP)

Aetiology

- Common in early pregnancy, therefore preterm birth
- Restriction of space and/or ability to turn due to:
    (i) firm abdominal and uterine muscles, e.g. primigravida
    (ii) uterine anomalies, e.g. fibroids; bicornuate

    (iii) oligohydramnios
    (iv) contracted pelvis
    (v) multiple pregnancy
    (vi) extended breech
- Excess space in uterus:
    - (i) lax abdominal and uterine muscles, e.g. grand(e) multiparity
    - (ii) polyhydramnios
- Fetal causes:
    - (i) hydrocephalus
    - (ii) IUD
    - (iii) IUGR and decreased fetal activity
    - (iv) short umbilical cord

Diagnosis

History

- Previous breech
- Maternal discomfort under ribs
- Fetal movements low in uterus

Abdominal palpation

- Not always easy, especially if breech deeply engaged/legs extended
- Presenting part feels less round, bony and ballottable
- Fundal part (head) hard, round and ballottable
- FH found above umbilicus (except when deeply engaged)

Ultrasound scan

X-ray

Vaginal examination in labour

- Presenting part may be high/soft
- Anal fissure, anus, sacrum may be felt (meconium on examining finger)

- Soft genitalia felt (difficult)
- Feet may be felt

Management – in pregnancy

- After 32–34 weeks, obstetric referral
- Promotion of spontaneous version (see Nevi *et al.* 2004)
    (i) moxibustion
    (ii) acupuncture
    (iii) knees–chest position
- 36 weeks – ? offer external cephalic version (ECV) (NICE 2008a)
- Persistent breech – decision on mode of delivery assisted by:
    (i) clinical judgement
    (ii) maternal wishes
    (iii) history
    (iv) fetal size, gestation, condition (US scan)
    (v) size, shape of pelvis (pelvimetry)

Mode of delivery

See Glazerman (2006) and Bewley and Shannon (2007) for **Breech Trial**
- Elective caesarean section common
- Spontaneous or assisted vaginal delivery; in urgent cases (see subsequent text) by a midwife (see *EU Second Midwifery Directive 80/155/EEC* in NMC 2004)

Management of labour

- Generally in hospital – senior obstetric supervision
- If at home (mother's informed choice) inform supervisor of midwives
- Anaesthetist/paediatrician on standby
- ? Induction of labour
- Continuous electronic monitoring usual
- Normal labour care

- Clear fluids orally (anaesthetic risk)
- ? Mobile (aids descent of breech) or bed rest (debatable)
- Usual analgesia (epidural prevents premature pushing and entrapment of fetal head in incompletely dilated cervix)
- Allow spontaneous rupture of membranes (VE to exclude cord prolapse)

Complications

- Pre-labour rupture of membranes
- Cord prolapse
- Genital tract bruising/oedema
- Placental separation in second stage
- Fetal hypoxia due to:
  - (i) cord compression
  - (ii) placental separation
  - (iii) inhalation of liquor, blood, mucus
- Entrapment of head in incompletely dilated cervix
- Undiagnosed CPD
- Intracranial haemorrhage due to:
  - (i) anoxia
  - (ii) tentorial tear
- Trauma from faulty handling, e.g.
  - (i) fractures
  - (ii) dislocations
  - (iii) muscle/nerve damage
  - (iv) ruptured abdominal organs
  - (v) perinatal mortality

Breech delivery

Part of a midwife's role in an emergency (NMC 2004); the midwife must remember the following points:
(i) medical aid – obstetrician/paediatrician
(ii) malpresentation means high risk of mortality/morbidity
(iii) ensure cervix is fully dilated
(iv) keep hands off the breech as much as possible
(v) ensure slow, controlled delivery of head

Aim

- Safe delivery of baby and placenta
- Minimise physical and psychological trauma for mother/baby

Preparation

- Explain breech delivery to mother
- Seek cooperation
- Ensure maternal bladder/rectum empty

Action

- Encourage mother to push
- Allow spontaneous delivery of buttocks
- Release legs as necessary
- When umbilicus is delivered, pull down cord loop, avoiding traction
- Allow weight of body to cause further descent
- Feel for/help deliver elbows/arms
- Wait for shoulders to rotate into antero-posterior diameter (use Løvset's manoeuvre if this fails to occur – see subsequent text)
- Grasp baby by iliac crests; tilt towards the maternal sacrum, releasing anterior shoulder
- Lift buttocks towards maternal abdomen, enabling posterior shoulder to deliver
- Allow the body to hang, enabling the head to flex; continue with Burns–Marshall manoeuvre (if the head remains deflexed, continue with Mauriceau–Smellie–Veit manoeuvre, i.e. jaw flexion and shoulder traction encourages head flexion)

Burns–Marshall manoeuvre

- When the hairline appears
- With a finger between the ankles keep the legs extended
- Take legs through 180° arc towards mother until mouth and nose appear at vulva
- Right hand guards perineum until head can be slowly delivered
- ? clear airways

Mauriceau–Smellie–Veit manoeuvre

- Straddle baby over the right arm, middle finger in baby's mouth
- Other fingers either side over the cheeks
- Left hand over baby's neck, middle finger splinting neck
- Other fingers over each shoulder
- Apply traction with right hand; push with left hand while head is slowly flexed
- When face free, deliver vault slowly

Løvset's manoeuvre

- Grasp baby by iliac crests
- Rotate body through half a circle with the back upwards
- Posterior shoulder to symphysis – shoulder and arm are freed
- Rotate body in reverse direction to release second shoulder and arm

Following delivery of the head

- Give Syntometrine (unless contraindicated)
- Cut cord, wrap baby, show to mother/take to Resuscitaire
- Deliver placenta/membranes (see **Delivery technique**, Management of third stage of labour)
- Observe for perineal trauma
- Carry out maternal/neonatal observations
- Contemporaneous records

Student activity

- Discover if ECV is performed in your unit and observe procedure
- Note local policies regarding management of labour
- Review birth register – how many breech deliveries conducted by midwives?
- Practice procedure using fetal doll and obstetric model/pelvis
- Further reading: Hannah *et al.* (2000); Nevi *et al.* (2004); NICE (2008a) (ECV); Westgren *et al.* (2005)

Brow presentation

See also **OP position** in Section 1.
 Head presenting midway between flexion and extension.

Diagnosis

Abdominal examination

- High presenting part
- Diameter of head may feel large
- ? Groove felt between head and back

Vaginal examination

- High presenting part possibly not felt
- Orbital ridges and anterior fontanelles felt

Ultasound scan

Management

- Emergency caesarean section – if the 13 cm mentovertical diameter enters the pelvic brim the head will arrest in the pelvic cavity. This is called obstructed labour
- Vaginal delivery if full head extension/flexion leads to face or vertex presentation

Caesarean section

- *Elective caesarean section*:
When vaginal delivery is not considered to be in the mother's / baby's best interests, e.g. in cases of cephalo-pelvic disproportion, placenta praevia, severe pre-eclampsia/PIH
- *Emergency caesarean section*:
When adverse conditions/emergency (e.g. cord prolapse) arise in labour – if anticipated, woman should be forewarned of possibility

Aim – pre-operative care

- Facilitate caesarean section delivery
- Support the woman/partner prn
- Ensure informed consent is gained in writing (NMC 2008)
- Assist obstetrician/paediatrician
- Ensure good recovery of mother/baby

Preparation – elective

- Locate/identify woman correctly – presence of ID band
- Check woman's understanding of procedures/operation – consent form signed with doctor
- Blood to laboratory for save serum/X-matching prn and clotting screening prn, e.g. in PIH/pre-eclampsia? Arrange a visit to NNU
- Ensure appropriate charts labelled
- Prescription sheet written up for premedication/post-operative analgesia
- Procedures:
    (i) woman fasted minimum of 6 hours prior to surgery
    (ii) antacids, skin preparation, bowel care given as policy
    (iii) bath/shower prior to surgery
    (iv) IV infusion sited prn
- Complete pre-op. checklist, e.g.:
    ○ Note:
        (i) blood results, i.e. ABO and Rh grouping, FBC and Hb, clotting screening prn
        (ii) observations, e.g. urinalysis, TPR and BP, FH/CTG
        (iii) allergies, e.g. drugs, metals, Elastoplast
        (iv) choice of baby names
        (v) dental bridges/caps present
        (vi) consent form signed
    ○ Remove:
        (i) dentures
        (ii) contact lens(es)
        (iii) jewellery – wedding ring may remain; cover with adhesive tape

(iv) make-up/nail polish

(v) hearing aid – ? removed after woman anaesthetised; to remain with her

Action

- Ask woman to empty bladder; catheter inserted under GA
- Give theatre gown/cap to put on
- Help with TED stockings prn (see Section 1)
- Follow special instructions
- Give premedication as prescribed; ensure safety whilst woman is under its influence
- Inform woman of estimated time of surgery
- Assist partner to prepare for theatre if attending delivery
- Escort to theatre
- Hand-over case records/other relevant documentation to theatre staff
- Pre-operative check list may be repeated

Preparation/action – emergency

- Pre-operative care minimal
- ? start MEWS/MOEWS chart
- Consent forms signed
- IV infusion sited
- Observations performed
- Support woman/partner; emergency caesarean section possibly a frightening experience
- Note choice of baby names
- Bladder emptied; catheter commonly inserted under GA
- NNU on standby

Immediate post-operative care

- Recovery from anaesthesia in operating theatre recovery area
- Close observation of:
    (i) airway/breathing – ? pulse oximetry for oxygen levels
    (ii) pulse and BP – ? continuous electronic monitoring

    (iii) blood loss *per vaginam*

    (iv) pain levels

    (v) levels of consciousness

- If spinal/epidural anaesthesia, mother usually alert, but still requires careful observation
- Mother/baby contact as soon as possible
- Inform/support partner
- Transferred to the ward when condition stable

Continued post-operative care

(NB: this is major abdominal surgery + uterine involution/reversal of pregnancy changes.)

- Ensure satisfactory post-operative recovery
- Give adequate analgesia
- Encourage development of mother–baby relationship
- Assist mother to achieve self-care/return to normal function
- Help with baby care/adjustment to motherhood

Preparation

- Bed prepared to receive post-operative client
- Observation charts/equipment (for IV infusion, urinary drainage bag/stands) prn
- Cot prepared
- Bell-call system accessible
- Ensure privacy

Action

- Receive woman/baby to ward
- Check identification labels
- Note special instructions
- Commence post-operative observations:

    (i) ? hourly pulse, blood pressure and respirations initially – then four hourly – ? continue MEWS/MOEWS chart

    (ii) palpate uterine fundus – ensure well contracted

(iii) wound for leakage

(iv) loss *per vaginam*

(v) urinary output/remove catheter as instructed

- Encourage leg movement/breathing exercises
- Ensure adequate analgesia – ? patient-controlled (PCA)/opiates IM 4–6 hourly
- Encourage ambulation as early as condition allows – adequate rest needed
- Assist with feeding baby
- Encourage contact with baby to promote a good relationship
- Offer support/advice prn
- If emergency caesarean section – ? de-briefing needed
- Normal postnatal care as mother recovers
- Accurate records

Student activity

Further reading: Hildingsson *et al.* (2003); Lilford *et al.* (2005); Smith *et al.* (2003).

Cardiotocography (CTG)

Simultaneous electronic monitoring of fetal heart and uterine contractions – recorded on special paper rotating at 1 cm per minute.

Types

External

Doppler ultrasound transducer on mother's abdomen (over most audible FH); pressure-sensitive transducer on maternal abdomen over uterine fundus.

Internal

- FSE on presenting part (breech/head) records ECG
- Intrauterine catheter (rarely used) records contractions

Indications for use

All 'high-risk' cases during pregnancy (periodic) and labour (continuous) (see NICE 2007).

Aims

Detection of fetal compromise, enabling prompt delivery and preventing fetal trauma – evidence/research about efficiency/benefits in labour inconclusive – much discussion about professionals' interpretative ability; also, is fetal distress in labour an indication of compromise *prior* to labour?

FH patterns

Normal baseline rate = 110–160 beats per minute (bpm)

Baseline variability = variation in rate over 10–20 seconds, i.e. 5–15 bpm

Accelerations = FH rate rises for 15 seconds in response to activity/stimulation, e.g. contractions, noise, application of FSE – 2 accelerations in 20 minutes = reactive trace and positive sign of fetal well-being

Baseline bradycardia = a persistent low rate >100 and <110 bpm, uncomplicated if without other indications – ensure recording is not of maternal origin; <100 bpm + other CTG/clinical indications = compromised fetus; caused by:

　(i) regional analgesia (epidural), especially if maternal hypotension

　(ii) congenital heart defects

　(iii) acute hypoxia during contraction, ? transient chemoreceptor-mediated bradycardia (or prolonged deceleration)

　(iv) excessive uterine activity

　(v) hypovolaemia following prolonged labour (usually mild)

　(vi) maternal hypotension due to:

　　– aortocaval compression (supine hypotension)

　　– epidural

　　– shock

Baseline tachycardia = persistently >160 bpm; uncomplicated unless other CTG or clinical indications
Caused by:

(i) fetal activity/stimulation, e.g. pain

(ii) prematurity <32–34 weeks

(iii) drugs to stop preterm labour

(iv) fetal anaemia, especially Rh isoimmunisation

(v) fetal bleeding, e.g. vessel puncture in amniocentesis, trauma in vasa praevia

(vi) following prolonged deceleration (in response to catecholamine production)

(vii) maternal pyrexia – infection; prolonged labour; epidural

(viii) maternal distress

(ix) maternal hyperthyroidism

Reduced variability (smooth trace) – 10 minute reduction insignificant (may be fetal sleep); observe for 40–50 minute period; but >180 minute = fetal acidosis, caused by:

(i) prematurity

(ii) maternal narcotic, sedative, antihypertensive, general anaesthetic

(iii) fetal hypoxia, e.g. in IUGR

(iv) placental insufficiency, e.g. due to multiple infarcts

(v) oxytocin – increased contractions may lower utero-placental perfusion

(vi) fetal malformation, e.g. CNS and heart

(vii) viral infection

However, cases of low variability have resulted in normal outcome
High variability = >25 bpm, caused by:

(i) external stimulation

(ii) cord compression and acute hypoxia

Early decelerations = a decrease in fetal heart rate before or at the beginning of a contraction; rapid return to normal after contraction caused by rapid progression in labour/descent of head due to:

(i) fetal head compression

(ii) raised intracranial pressure and vagal nerve response

Late decelerations = decreased rate after onset of contraction with lowest point after peak of contraction = fetal compromise; caused by:

(i) uteroplacental insufficiency

(ii) fetal hypoxia

Variable decelerations = variable in timing, frequency and depth; usually short duration; may/may not indicate acute hypoxia (depending on length and depth); caused by:

(i) cord compression

(ii) pressure over orbital ridges, e.g. in breech, posterior position, CPD

Physiology of variable decelerations in healthy fetus:

(i) As cord compresses, vein compresses first; BP falls; this stimulates baroreceptors in autonomic nervous system, so FH goes up

(ii) Cord arteries then compress; increased pressure stimulates baroreceptors; then FH falls

(iii) As artery pressure comes off, FH rises above normal

(iv) As all pressure comes off, FH returns to normal

Sinusoidal pattern = the cause of this pattern is not fully understood but presents as a regular undulating waveform above and below normal baseline rate – 2–5 cycles per minute; absent short-term variability and reactivity; may be typical or atypical, caused by:

(i) absent neural control of heart

(ii) brain stem hypoxia

(iii) fetal anaemia – Rh isoimmunisation; fetal bleeding; feto-maternal haemorrhage

(iv) severe hypoxia

(v) thumb sucking (seen on scan); pattern only short-term

Discussion

Clinical situation *must* be considered along with CTG, e.g.

(i) history – general and obstetric

(ii) maternal condition – general, antenatal, intrapartum

(iii) gestation (<28 weeks; FH variations are unreliable; immature fetal autonomic nervous system)

(iv) uterine contractions, labour stage and progress

(v) clear/meconium liquor

(vi) fetal blood sample

Student activity

• Revise the mechanism of heart rate control

• Note your local policy on antenatal and intrapartum CTG use

• Familiarise yourself with your unit equipment

• Some students use the mnemonic Dr C Bravado to remember main points when looking at fetal heart recordings: Dr = determine risk, C = contractions, Bra = basal rate, v = variability, a = acceleration, d = decelerations, o = overall assessment (American Academy of Family Physicians 2005)

• Further reading: NICE 2007

Carpal tunnel syndrome

Signs and symptoms

'Pins and needles'/numbness in the fingers.

Aetiology

• Local oedema compressing median nerve in carpal tunnel at the wrist

• Usually resolves postnatally as oedema subsides

Management

• If severe, physiotherapist referral

• Exercises/supporting splint

Catheterisation

Aim

Empty the bladder with minimum discomfort

Leave the catheter *in situ* prn

Preparation

- Clean area to work on
- Catheterisation pack
- Appropriate-sized catheter – narrow lumen if in labour
- Sterile gloves
- Cleansing solution
- Ampoule of sterile water and syringe if indwelling catheter
- Local anaesthetic gel may be used
- Urinary drainage bag, specimen bottle prn
- Ensure privacy, seek consent, explain procedure

Action

- Aseptic technique (see preceding text) – use sterile gloves
- Protect the bed, open pack, apply gloves
- Swab vulva
- Local anaesthetic gel may be applied to end of catheter
- Separate labia, locate urethra (not always easy in labour; aim 2.5 cm below clitoris)
- Insert catheter gently into urethra – ? as much as 10 cm in labour (fetal head may interfere with catheter passage)
- Collect urine into receiver and measure – ? collect specimen for laboratory
- Remove catheter or fill balloon with sterile water and connect to closed drainage system if catheter is indwelling
- Make woman comfortable
- Accurate records

Cephalo-pelvic disproportion (CPD)

Aetiology

- Large fetus, e.g. genetic origin/maternal diabetes
- Small pelvis – ? woman of small stature
- Abnormal pelvis:
  - (i) non-gynaecoid shape
  - (ii) disease, e.g. rickets/osteomalacia

(iii) fracture, e.g. road accident
(iv) spinal deformity
• Malposition, e.g. occipito-posterior

Considerations for diagnosis – during pregnancy

• Non-engaged fetal head in primigravida at 38 weeks/multigravida at term
• Abnormal presentation, e.g. breech
• Previous prolonged/difficult labour/delivery

Considerations for diagnosis – during labour

• Head slow to progress in labour, i.e.
  (i) slow/halted cervical dilatation
  (ii) head advancement slow in second stage – ? deep transverse arrest (DTA) – (see **OP position** in Section 1)
• Hypertonic uterine action and severe pain
• Hypotonic uterus, i.e. contractions start well, then slow/halt inco-ordinate uterine action
• Excess moulding of fetal skull
• Large caput formation
• Bandl's (retraction) ring formed

Management – in pregnancy

• Obstetric referral
• X-ray pelvimetry (fetal head and maternal pelvis measured on X-ray film)
• Assess CPD degree – if major, elective caesarean section; if minor, ? trial of labour

Management – in labour

• Medical aid
• Continuous fetal monitoring
• Maternal condition closely monitored:
  (i) vital signs
  (ii) urine output and urinalysis

- Change maternal position/mobilise
- Adequate analgesia, and discontinue Syntocinon if uterus hyper-tonic
- Consider using Syntocinon if uterus hypotonic
- ? Instrumental delivery
- Emergency caesarean section if fetal/maternal compromise

Complications

- Obstructed labour
- Cord prolapse
- Instrumental/operative delivery
- Ruptured uterus
- Perinatal morbidity/death and maternal morbidity or (in developing countries) death

Student activity

- Revise the pelvis
- Further reading: Connolly *et al*. (2003)

Changing Childbirth

(DH 1993).

A Government expert maternity group's response (chair Baroness Cumberledge) to the Winterton Report (1992), proposing radical changes in maternity services. Woman-centred, appropriate, accessible and effective care, to be facilitated by women's choices and control in care provision. Consumer satisfaction to be aided by continuity in professional care. Many units now offer a team midwifery approach to improve continuity; some offer case-load care.

Student activity

- Consider your unit's service provision in the light of *Changing Childbirth* (DH 1993). Compare this to *Maternity Matters* (DH 2007a)
- Further reading: Hicks *et al*. (2003)

Child protection

Legal protection contained in the Children Act 1989 (with consequent Rules of Court Regulations and Guidelines) provides the framework for state and voluntary agencies to work together to prevent children suffering harm from their carers. Local social services departments must ensure the welfare of children when they are away from their parents – e.g. in children's homes, nurseries, foster placements, boarding schools or hospitals. *Working Together to Safeguard Children: A Guide to Inter-agency Working to Safeguard and Promote the Welfare of Children* (Dcsf 2006) is a key document for any professional working in the field of child protection. Hospital Trusts have local policies and guidance for child protection – e.g. for recognition of abuse, protocols for dealing with suspected abuse, agencies to contact, case conference procedures and record keeping. The child may be put on the Child Protection Register or may be made the subject of a case order. The child has a say in the proceedings.

Student activity

Further reading: Reder and Duncan (2003).

The Children Act, 1989

Reviewed in the Adoption and Children Act 2002 and the Children and Adoption Act 2006, the Act includes both private and public law, e.g. what happens to children after divorce and the responsibilities of the Social Service Department (SSD). Family Law Courts deal with issues of residency following divorce and Youth Courts with young offenders.

Main principles

- Welfare of the child is paramount
- Children should remain with their own families wherever possible

• Parents retain responsibility for their children, even if no longer living with them
• SSD gives appropriate help to parents of children in need
• Children should live in a safe environment, with effective intervention if they are in danger
• Children should be kept informed/participate in decisions about their future
• Following adoption children may have contact with birth parents if seen to be in their best interest

Cholestasis

Impaired maternal liver: a rarely diagnosed, possibly under-diagnosed condition.

Aetiology

• Unclear
• Commoner in multiple pregnancies
• ? High oestrogen levels
• ? Genetic origin

Signs and symptoms

• General pruritus (itching) in late pregnancy, often starting in hands/feet
• Occasionally jaundice
• Dark urine
• Steatorrhoea (*ste-at-o-rea*) (undigested fat in faeces)
• Raised serum bile acids/liver enzymes

Management

• Senior obstetrician referral (urgent)
• Hepatologist referral
• FBC; clotting screening
• Prophylactic maternal vitamin K
• Relieve itching locally, e.g. with calamine lotion

- Induced preterm delivery
- Continuous fetal monitoring in labour
- IVI *in situ*
- Prepare for possible PPH

Student activity

Further reading: Coombes (2000); Greenes and Williamson (2009).

Chorionic Villus Sampling (CVS)

Not a midwife's procedure; carried out transcervically at 6–13 weeks (commonly 8–9 weeks) using ultrasound.

Aim

Aseptically remove chorionic villi (placental tissue) for investigation.

Preparation

- Full explanation of procedure to woman
- Consent obtained (NMC 2008) (? counselling previously)
- Dressing trolley prepared
- Appropriate packs/equipment prn
- Detailed scan; confirms gestation, viability, excludes multiple pregnancy

Action

- Woman made comfortable in lithotomy position
- Assist by opening packs/equipment
- Doctor – thoroughly cleanses thighs, vulva, cervix to minimise risk of infection
- Malleable cannula bent to required shape and introduced into cervical canal under USS guidance
- Aspiration using a syringe/vacuum pump achieves placental biopsy
- Sample placed into appropriate container, labelled, sent to laboratory

• Woman made comfortable/allowed to rest until ready to go home
• Advised to ring hospital if complications arise and for test results
• Procedure recorded in woman's records

Student activity

Consider advantages/disadvantages of CVS compared to amniocentesis.

CLAPA

(The Cleft Lip and Palate Association)

A national support agency based in London, with local groups offering information, advice and support to parents with a baby with cleft lip and/or palate.

1st Floor, Green Man Tower,
332B Goswell Road,
London EC1V 7LQ.
Tel: 0171 824 8110.
Fax: 020 7833 5999
Email: info@clapa.com
http://www.clapa.com

Clasp trial

A Collaborative Low-dose Aspirin Study in Pregnancy.

Method

A randomised, placebo, double-blind trial conducted in 213 centres in 16 countries between January 1988 and December 1992 evaluating daily low-dose aspirin in the prevention/treatment of pre-eclampsia. Over 9000 women between 12 and 32 weeks pregnant with a high risk/signs of pre-eclampsia/IUGR took part. Half had 60 mg aspirin daily, the rest a placebo (dummy). Both women and professionals were unaware which was being taken (double blind).

Results

• 12% reduction in proteinuric pre-eclampsia (statistically not significant) (Every 1994)
• Reduced risk of early-onset pre-eclampsia (APEC 1994)
• Does not prevent IUGR (APEC 1994)
• One-quarter reduced risk of severe pre-eclampsia (suggested by a meta-analysis, i.e. combining this trial with others) (APEC 1994)

Cleft lip and palate

A congenital condition, either separate or together – 'split' in upper lip and/or in hard palate (mouth roof) or soft palate (back of mouth).

Diagnosis

Part of the midwife's initial examination of the newborn (NB: soft palate cleft easily missed).

Management

• Sensitively inform parents
• Promote parent–infant attachment (distressing condition)
• Paediatric and surgical referral
• Aids to feeding – cup/spoon (see **Cup feeding**):
   (i) individually made dental plate fitting roof of the baby's mouth
   (ii) special teat
• Repair of cleft lip usually in early weeks after birth – often several operations
• Repair of cleft palate when a few months old – often several operations
• Referral to support group CLAPA (see the previous entry)

Student activity

Note your local procedure for congenital cleft lip/palate.

Clinical governance

As directed in the Government White Paper *The New NHS – Modern, Dependable* (DH 1997), Trusts have accountability for clinical governance, with practitioners accepting responsibility for developing and maintaining clinical standards. Overseeing local processes is the Commission for Health Improvement (CHIMP), while the National Institute for Health and Clinical Excellence (NICE) gives national guidelines on services and clinical cost-effectiveness.

Student activity

Further reading: Currie *et al.* (2003).

Centre for Maternal and Child Enquiries (CMACE)

Registered charity set up in July 2009 with Baroness Julia Cumberledge as patron.

Aim

To improve the health of mothers, babies and children by carrying out confidential enquiries and related work on a nationwide basis and by widely disseminating findings and recommendations (encompasses CEMACH – see subsequent entry); http://www.cmace.org.uk.

Community Health Councils (CHCs)

Independent, statutory bodies originally set up by Government in 1974, they formed a link between service providers and users, with a legal duty to represent the consumers' interests. Primary Care Trusts (PCTs) have taken over this function, and patient advisory liaison services (PALS) provide for consumer interest.

Complementary therapies

Treatment/therapy that replaces, complements or enhances orthodox medicine.

Types

- *Acupressure*:

Similar to acupuncture, but using finger pressure

- *Acupuncture*:

Traditional Chinese therapy – fine needles inserted into the skin stimulate nerve pathways, influencing other parts of the body and often offering pain relief

- *Aromatherapy*:

Essential oils extracted from plants or flowers (neat or mixed with a base) – vapours inhaled, applied as a compress, ingested, added to bath water – e.g. aiding relaxation

- *Chiropractic*:

Manipulation of spine

- *Herbalism*:

Medication from plant materials – taken orally, added to the bath, applied to the skin

- *Homeopathy*:

A holistic treatment using like to cure like – natural substances (e.g. plants, seeds, metals, insects) given orally in very dilute solutions

- *Hydrotherapy*:

Use of water for exercise, relaxation or pain relief, e.g. aquanatal exercises and water births

- *Hypnotherapy*:

Hypnosis, i.e. induced relaxation and auto-suggestion to control body activity or aid coping mechanism

- *Massage*:

Rubbing and kneading of the body for relaxation or pain relief (midwives know that back rubbing relieves labour pain)

- *Meditation*:

Deep reflection; may be accompanied by relaxation techniques

- *Music/sound therapy*:

Soothing music aids relaxation; uterine sounds may aid baby's sleep

- *Osteopathy*:

Joint manipulation

- *Psychoprophylaxis*:

Combination of breathing exercises and relaxation techniques aids coping with labour (see **Relaxation techniques**)

- *Physiotherapy*:

Muscular exercise to improve muscle tone/joint mobility/circulation

- *Reflexology*:

Massage of specific points in hands or feet to stimulate the energy (nerve) pathways influencing other parts of the body

- *Relaxation techniques*:

To relax mind and body (see also separate categories)

- *Shiatsu*:

A Japanese development from Chinese medicine; simple pressure, holding techniques and gentle stretching influence nerve pathways

- *T.E.N.S.*:

Transcutaneous (via the skin) electric nerve stimulation; low-powered electricity via small skin pads stimulates nerves, blocking pain sensations' access to cerebral cortex

- *Yoga*:

A Hindu method of exercise and discipline promoting physical and spiritual well-being

Dangers/contraindications in childbearing

- Joint manipulation may damage lax joints
- Some herbal or aromatherapy substances are toxic/harmful to the mother/fetus
- Some therapies alter BP (up or down), others uterine action (implications for progress in labour/fetal or maternal compromise)
- 'Emergency' conditions/situations may be missed or inappropriately managed

Professional accountability

- A midwife must have a midwifery-appropriate qualification before practising and adhere to local policies and guidelines (NMC 2004) and medicine administration (NMC 2007)

• Consider insurance (personal/vicarious); record keeping (NMC 2009)

Student activity

• Note your local policies on complementary therapies, aquanatal and waterbirth
• Essential reading: *Midwives' Rules and Standards* (NMC 2004), *Standards for Medicines Management* (NMC 2007)
• Further reading: Dimond (2006); Tiran and Mack (2000)

Confidential Enquiry into Maternal and Child Health (CEMACH)

See **CMACE**.

CEMACH is the successor to CEMD and CESDI, launched in 2003. It is a self-governing body funded by the National Institute of Clinical Excellence (NICE). Enquiries continue into maternal, perinatal and infant deaths and will be extended to encompass morbidity and a national enquiry into child health. The board has members from the Royal College of Obstetricians and Gynaecologists, Royal College of Midwives, Royal College of Paediatrics and Child Health, Royal College of Pathologists, Royal College of Anaesthetists and Faculty of Health, with extensive lay and voluntary sector involvement. Online: http://www.cemach.org.uk/.

Confidential Enquiry into Maternal Deaths (CEMD)

It is a series of triennial (3-yearly) reports that began in 1952, then covering England and Wales, but now the whole of the United Kingdom. A team of specialists audit all maternal deaths to identify causes and trends. Recommendations are often made by the team for 'best practice' in specific situations to prevent future deaths. Now an integral part of **CEMACH**.

Confidential Enquiry into Stillbirths and Deaths in Infancy (CESDI)

CESDI began in 1992; data have been collected since 1993 related to infant and perinatal mortality via a rapid reporting system. Now an integral part of **CEMACH**.

Congenital dislocation of hips

Abnormal development of one/both hip joints present at birth, with partial/complete displacement of femur head from acetabulum.

Aetiology

- Approximately 1:1500 births
- Genetic in origin; commoner in females/within families
- Intrauterine position, i.e. commoner in breech/oligohydramnious cases

Diagnosis

- During routine neonatal screening (midwife/paediatrician)
- Barlow's or Ortolani's test
- Ultrasound scan

Management

- Paediatric referral
- Orthopaedic referral
- Splint to flex and abduct hips; 3 months continuous wear promotes joint formation

Complications – if undiagnosed

- Difficulty/inability walking
- Leg shortening
- Prolonged treatment; ? surgery

Student activity

Note local screening method (when/by whom).

CONI (care of next infant)

A programme of support, set up by the Foundation for the Study of Infant Deaths (FSID), for families where a previous baby has died. A multidisciplinary approach is used, with local co-ordinators offering help, information and support as required during pregnancy and following childbirth (see **Stillbirth**).

Contraception advice

Offered postnatally; individually timed for woman/couple's needs/ wishes; cultural/religious beliefs influence acceptability. Sexual inter-course may be commenced as soon as the mother is comfortable; caution – potential maternal deaths due to air embolism.

Keys to contraceptive advice

- Effective communication
- Non-judgemental approach
- Confidentiality
- Offered in privacy
- Up-to-date information, including availability
- Timing/method acceptable to individual/couple

Methods available	*Advice*
Barrier methods:	
(i) Male/female condom	(i) Use at any time
	No-petroleum lubricant, e.g. Vaseline, in place before any genital contact

(ii) Diaphragm (cap)	(ii) Used with spermicide In place before any genital contact; remains in place minimum 6 hours Existing cap size no longer right; fit/re-fit 6 weeks PN
(iii) Spermicides – creams, gels, foam, pessaries	(iii) Not effective alone

Hormonal:

(i) Combined oestrogen and progesterone pill/patch	(i) Unsuitable if breastfeeding, high BP, or smoker >35 Start 3 weeks PN – safe immediately; if later, add second method for 7 days; 12-hour safety time (if pill missed); if any later add second method for 7 days. Pill not safe if diarrhoea, vomiting, or with use of certain antibiotics; add second method for 7 days after episode
(ii) Progesterone only (mini pill)	(ii) Suitable when combined pill is not Start 3 weeks PN, safe immediately If later start, use second method for 7 days 3-hour safety time if pill missed – if any later, use second method for 7 days Not safe if diarrhoea, vomiting; add second method for 7 days after episode. Unaffected by antibiotics

(iii) Progesterone, IM (slow release)

(iii) ? Delayed return of fertility
? Menstrual irregularities
Start fifth day PN, safe immediately
Start after 6 weeks if BF, and also use second method for 7 days
Repeat every 12 weeks (Depo-Provera)
Repeat every 8 weeks (Noristat)

(iv) Progesterone implants:

(iv) 1 capsule implanted under skin (Implanon) of upper arm (slow release)
Insert 21 days PN; safe immediately
If inserted any later, also use second method for 7 days
Replace 5-yearly

(v) Progesterone intrauterine system (e.g. Mirena) (slow release)

(v) Hormone-impregnated coil
Insert 6 weeks PN, safe immediately
Replace 3 yearly

Intrauterine contraceptive device (IUCD) (coil):

Insert 6 weeks PN; safe immediately
Replace 3–5 yearly
First 2–3 periods ? heavy/painful

Natural family planning:

Acceptable in certain religions/cultures
Needs knowledge/motivation
Needs specialist teaching

Emergency contraception:

After unprotected intercourse/failed contraceptive method

(i) Hormonal (Schering PC4)	(i) High progesterone tabs. within 72 hours Available from family planning clinics, GP, some A and E departments, pregnancy advisory clinics and pharmacists
(ii) IUCD	(ii) Inserted within 5 days after intercourse or within 5 days after ovulation Available at family planning clinics, some GPs
Sterilisation: (i) Female tubal ligation	(i) Usually after 12 weeks PN General anaesthetic/hospital stay Safe immediately NHS/private hospital
(ii) Male vasectomy	(ii) Performed at any time Unsafe until three semen specimens sperm-free – may take several weeks Local/general anaesthetic – day care NHS (waiting list)/private hospital
? Future	perhaps a male 'pill'

Student activity

- Identify local family planning clinics – times and locations
- Consider the needs of teenagers, specific religious/ethnic groups
- Further reading: Family Planning Association website http://www.fpa.org.uk

Convulsions

See **Eclampsia**, **Epilepsy** and **Jittery baby**.

Cord prolapse/presentation

• Prolapse – cord loop presents following membrane rupture
• Presentation – cord loop lies below presenting part, membranes intact (occult if unseen/felt at side)

Aetiology

• Long cord increases risk
• Poorly fitting presenting part in maternal pelvis, e.g.:
    (i)   malpresentation, e.g. breech (especially footling); shoulder
    (ii) malposition, e.g. occipito-posterior
    (iii) small fetus, e.g. preterm labour
    (iv) high presenting part – especially at membrane rupture
    (v)   CPD, e.g. abnormal maternal pelvis; large baby
    (vi) multiple pregnancy
    (vii) uterine fibroids
    (viii) placenta praevia

Diagnosis

• Pregnancy – USS
• Labour:
    (i) VE
    (ii) suspected in certain CTG patterns

Management

See Figures 4 and 5.

Complications

• Fetal hypoxia due to:
    (i) cord compression
    (ii) vessel spasm from cooling/drying/handling

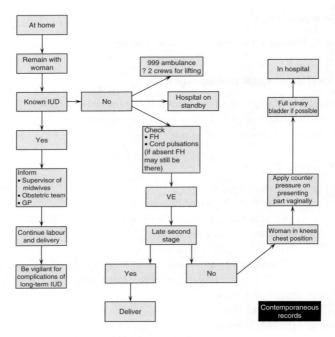

Figure 4 Cord prolapse – presentation at home.

- Birth asphyxia
- Long-term consequences of hypoxia/asphyxia
- Perinatal death
- Surgical intervention for mother; immediate/long-term risks
- Psychological trauma/post-traumatic stress

Student activity

- Note your local policy/procedures
- Further reading: Murphy and MacKenzie (2005)

Cramp

Painful muscle spasms – usually legs.

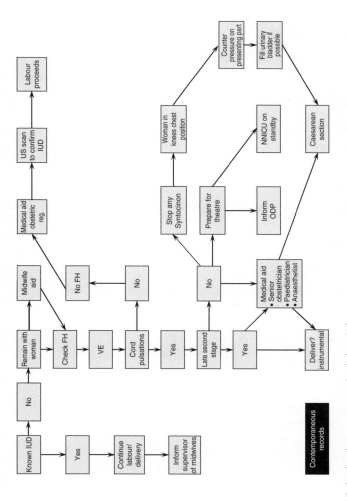

Figure 5 Cord prolapse – presentation in hospital.

Aetiology

Common in pregnancy – cause unproven.

Management

Massage and dorsiflexion of leg (pointing toes towards knee).

Crying baby

Causes

- Hunger
- Pain – wind, colic, trauma, illness
- Wrong temperature – too hot/cold
- Uncomfortable – position, soiled nappy
- Lonely, frightened, bored, startled

Management

Identify cause

- ? Obvious – feed time/rooting reflex; known trauma/illness
- Thorough history from mother/records

Observe baby's

- General well-being/condition:
    - (i) urine output
    - (ii) stool colour, consistency, frequency
    - (iii) skin colour/tone
- General behaviour:
    - (i) state of alertness
    - (ii) rapid leg movements ? indicate wind/colic
    - (iii) cry type – shrill sound ? cerebral irritation/pain
    - (iv) cry onset – sudden noise; dark/quiet ? fear/loneliness
    - (v) cry ceasing – when spoken to/nursed (relieves boredom)
    - (vi) eagerness to feed

- Environment:
  - (i) clothing/bedding
  - (ii) room temperature

Thorough examination

- Temperature and heart rate
- State of fontanelle
- Muscle tone and reflexes

Consider

- Feed type, frequency, amount
- Breastfeeding mother's fluid/nutritional intake
- Correct preparation, storage, feeding technique of formula

Provide

- Appropriate information/advice
- Promotion of mother's confidence – encouragement/support
- Medical aid prn

Cultural aspects related to childbirth

Culture – a way of life (values, beliefs, conduct). Reproduction, menstruation, fertility and sexuality are sensitive issues surrounded by customs, religious practices, folk beliefs, taboos. Pregnancy/parenthood may have many different meanings – you do not have to share other people's beliefs to provide care sympathetically. These points are a *guide* only, as everyone is individual and may not follow these customs. Always ask what the individual wishes. Non-British naming systems may present difficulties in addressing individuals and record-keeping.

Pregnancy

- A transition period – often viewed as dangerous
- Modesty may make examination difficult/only acceptable by another woman

- Woman may be accompanied by husband or son, only communicating through him (not just a language problem)
- Husband's permission may have to be sought before treatment/care given
- Rules may govern workload during pregnancy – often reduced or stopped by specific weeks

Childbirth

- May be viewed as natural, supernatural, a duty, an illness, a normal physiological process, a private or social event, a sexual experience
- In biblical times associated with punishment for sins of Eve; therefore pain and sorrow essential
- Choice of analgesia and expression of pain may be culturally determined (Queen Victoria's use of chloroform in 1853 for a pain-free labour initiated acceptance of pain relief for labour in the United Kingdom)

Menstruation and the postnatal period

- Women may be viewed as unclean, dangerous, polluting, magical, spiritual, powerful; they may be isolated physically, with certain restrictions, e.g. no hair-washing, swimming, sexual contact/physical contact with men
- Rules on bed rest/confinement, diet, re-introduction to family, ritual cleansing (i.e. physically and spiritually)
- Social status may be changed
- Rules on return to work may apply

Fetal/baby's rights

Stage of attainment of human status varies – this influences rules regarding:
(i) abortion
(ii) stillbirth burial
(iii) infant naming
(iv) infant-rearing practices

Ceremonies for baby

• Bathing may/may not be acceptable
• Circumcision
• Naming – several days/months later
• Baptism
• Specific rules for stillbirth, e.g. who can touch the baby, disposal of the body, agreement to post-mortem

Infant feeding

• Method of feeding may have social, symbolic or economic meaning
• Breastfeeding may be delayed until all colostrum expressed (seen as poison)
• Breastfeeding may be acceptable in public or only privately
• Dietary rules on what can be eaten may apply during breastfeeding

Role of men

• Varies from total avoidance/physical contact to close intimacy
• New Guinea husbands must 'build' the fetus and 'feed' the uterus with semen
• Presence at delivery ranges from taboo to expected
• Ritual *couvade* – men go through sympathetic labour in another place

Chinese culture, diet/rituals

• May be Christian, Muslim or Buddhist
• Good manners and politeness important
• Woman may wish female professional
• Open declaration of emotion may not be acceptable; may express social or psychological problems as physical symptoms, e.g. pain in an organ (NB: danger that depression is missed or misdiagnosed)
• Believe in balance of *Yin* (cold principle) and *Yang* (hot principle) by use of appropriate food or medication – meat, eggs, rice, wine, gaseous drinks, spicy foods, iron and vitamin tablets are 'hot'; bland, low-fat foods, vegetables, fruit, milk and milk products are cold; rice, fish and noodles are neutral

- Some illnesses/conditions are hot, e.g. pregnancy; or cold, e.g. menstruation and puerperium
- Postnatally isolated in one room, unable to eat with the family, or wash hair, dishes or clothes; cold water/wind, e.g. fan or open window, to be avoided
- Baby's 'hot' or 'cold' condition influences maternal diet when breastfeeding
- Baby not bathed for 3 days
- Official birth celebration at 1 month

Hindu culture, diet/rituals

- Avoid meat, especially beef; eggs may/may not be eaten (implications for medicines)
- Caste system (social class) strictly recognised
- Relatives visit for prayer within 4 days of birth
- 40 days postnatal rest

Jehovah's Witness – beliefs

- A Christian group who believe, for Bible-based reasons, that they must refuse blood or blood products, e.g. plasma (alternatives acceptable); anti-D immunoglobulin
- Possible difficulties when APH or PPH occur or in Rhesus-negative women

Read your local policy and procedures as to when blood products are refused

Further reading: Liston (2007); Muramoto (2001)

Jewish – diet/rituals

- Food must be *Kosher*, i.e. specifically prepared, ritually accepted; no pork/shellfish
- Sabbath (dusk Friday to dusk Saturday) restricts activities, e.g. switching on light
- Women modest, ? inform children/family of pregnancy (no AN home visit – confidentiality)

- Husband may sit in labour room/nearby, reading prayers: no physical contact
- Bed rest taken for 10 days postnatally (NB: prevention of DVT)
- Postnatally/during menstruation (unclean) – for set time husbands avoid physical contact
- Breastfeeding is the norm
- Male circumcision by a highly trained expert (may be a Rabbi) on the eighth day

Muslim culture, diet/rituals

- Follow religion of Islam
- Food *Halal*, i.e. specifically prepared, i.e. lawful/permitted; honey and dried prunes religious food; no pork or alcohol (implications for medication)
- *Ramadan* (1 month of fasting from dawn to dusk): diabetics and breastfeeding women are exempt, but pregnant women are not (they may not comply)
- May not discuss intimate topics through husband or son when acting as interpreter
- Modesty may mean a female professional must attend
- Pain of labour accepted without analgesia
- All male babies circumcised
- Baby's head shaved at birth/within 14 days
- Colostrum may be expressed and not given to baby
- A call to prayer whispered into baby's ear by father/religious person soon after birth
- Outward grief suppressed if stillbirth

Sikh culture, rituals/diet

- No beef, possibly vegetarian (implications for some medication)
- Women comparatively outgoing/ ? woman doctor
- Forty days postnatal rest

Student activity

Further reading: Bifulco (2004); Hillier (2003) (see reading related to Jehovah's Witness above).

Cup feeding

Aim

Provide an alternative method of giving breast milk (or formula milk) to babies who are unable or too weak/immature to suck.

Preparation

- Expressed breast milk/formula milk in sterile container
- Explain procedure to mother
- Baby clean/comfortable
- Sterile medicine cup (or similar) for giving feed
- Feeding chart labelled

Action

- Hold baby securely; upright position, maintaining eye contact
- Place a few millilitres of milk into cup
- Place the cup just touching lower lip; tip it, allowing baby to lap milk with its tongue
- Leaving cup in position during the feed allows baby to control own intake
- Observe baby carefully, ensuring no problems swallowing
- Refill cup prn, noting amount taken each time
- Allow plenty of time for feed
- Following feed, settle baby comfortably
- Record intake accurately on feeding chart
- Wash cup thoroughly prior to re-sterilising it

Student activity

Further reading: Trotter (2006).

Cystic fibrosis

See **Heel prick** and **Neonatal screening**.

Genetic defect; affects chloride transportation across membranes; secretions become sticky; affects pancrease (with malabsorption), lungs (chest infections); male infertility; reduced life span (approximately 31 years).

Incidence: (varies across United Kingdom).

- 1:2500 cases annually in the United Kingdom
- 1:25 of population carriers (UKNSPC 2007)

Student activity

- Ascertain your local policy for screening, and support services for parents of an affected child
- Further reading: *UK Newborn Screening Programme Centre* (UKNSPC 2008). Online: http://www.newbornbloodspot.screening.nhs.uk/

Cystitis

Bladder inflammation – untreated ? progress to severe UTI/septicaemia.

Aetiology

Commonly bacterial, often *Escherichia coli* organism (normal bowel flora).

Signs and symptoms

- Stinging/burning on micturition (PU)
- Lower abdominal discomfort/pain
- Pyrexia (high temperature)
- General malaise (feel unwell)

Investigations

See **Urinary tract infection – UTI**.

Management

- Copious oral fluids
- Appropriate medication

- Good hygiene minimises recurrence
- Tissue cleansing from front to back avoids anal contamination
- Regular/complete bladder emptying (problematic during pregnancy)
- Emptying bladder following sexual intercourse

Deep vein thrombosis

Also see **Embolism**.

Thrombosis (clot formation) in a deep vein; commonly, lower leg; iliac or femoral veins; (may result in thromboembolism).

Risk factors

- Immobility, e.g. bed rest; operative delivery
- Previous history of thromboembolic disorder
- Obesity
- Smoking
- Increases with age

Prevention

- Avoid immobility – during labour/postnatally
- Anticoagulants, e.g. heparin – if major risk (Drife 2007)
- TED stockings (see Section 1) if identified risk
- Avoid dehydration
- No oestrogen, as in, e.g. combined oral contraception

Signs and symptoms

- ? Asymptomatic
- Slight pyrexia/slight tachycardia
- Lower abdominal, groin, calf pain, depending on clot location
- Leg ? oedematous, pale, cooler

Diagnosis

- History
- Clot location by USS/venography (X-ray following injection of dye into veins)

Management

- See Drife (2007)
- Medical aid
- Anticoagulants – IV heparin – bolus dose and/or in an intravenous infusion or SC heparin
- Blood for clotting screening
- Bed rest – ? elevate foot of bed; use a bed cradle
- Analgesics
- Observe for abnormal bleeding, e.g. lochia/wounds; general condition; vital signs
- Anticoagulants continued after discharge – usually orally, i.e. heparin in pregnancy/warfarin postnatal

Complications

- Potentially life threatening – moving clot (embolism) lodges elsewhere – commonly lung (pulmonary embolism) or brain (cerebral embolism)
- Thromboembolic conditions are the highest cause of direct maternal deaths in the United Kingdom (see Drife 2007)

Delivery technique

As independent, accountable practitioners, midwives develop individual views on childbirth management. Partnership in care/choices in position for birth mean that prescriptive delivery techniques are no longer feasible. However, principles of safe delivery that apply for home and hospital are included here.

Aim

- Deliver the baby safely
- Minimise harm to both mother and/or baby
- Early detection/management of deviations from normal
- Reduce the risk of postnatal infection
- Accommodate woman's/partner's wishes in achieving a satisfactory/fulfilling outcome

Preparation

• Vaginal delivery can only be a clean (rather than an aseptic) procedure; however, all preparations as for aseptic technique
• Delivery pack/instruments
• Cleansing solution (note local policy) – warmed if possible
• Syntometrine prepared for IM injection prn (NB: prepared by the practitioner administering)
• Ensure warm environment/cot
• Identification bands for newborn in hospital; (see **Identification of newborn at birth**)
• Other equipment to aid woman's choice of position, e.g. wedges, bean bags, cushions
• Discussion with woman previously about any special wishes, e.g. partner to cut cord
• Position yourself on mother's right (depending on birth position adopted)

Action

• Directed pushing (Valsalva manoeuvre) unnecessary in the light of research; however, woman may value midwife's instruction, particularly as head is crowning
• Spontaneous pushing encouraged
• Delivery pack opened/equipment prepared once progress is being made (timing depends on parity/position)
• Sterile gloves/protective clothing worn
• Vulva/perineum swabbed, drapes on bed/floor (depends on birth position)

Delivery of head in occipito-anterior position

• Allow head to advance with maternal effort
• As head distends perineum, apply pressure with left cupped hand to prevent rapid delivery/perineal trauma (see **HOOP study**) (flexing the head of doubtful value)
• As the head crowns, woman asked not to push but pant/breathe Entonox to facilitate slow delivery

• Once the biparietal diameter has delivered, head is eased out by extension
• Whilst awaiting restitution/external rotation, feel neck for cord (*some controversy about this and next cord points*)
• If cord present and loose – a loop can be freed by pulling over the head
• If cord present and very tight, medical aid; try to deliver baby without cutting cord; if impossible, apply two artery forceps, cut between, release cord
• When shoulders rotate, encourage woman to push with the next contraction; midwife guides the baby's head towards the perineum, allowing delivery of anterior shoulder
• Syntometrine commonly given IM by an assistant at this point
• Baby's head is eased towards the symphysis, releasing posterior shoulder
• Baby is supported beneath the axillae; body delivered towards mother's abdomen (NB: check that direct skin-to-skin contact is acceptable)
• Apgar score is assessed
• Cord commonly cut at this point (but see **Third-stage management**)
• Dry baby and observe onset of respirations
• Mother–baby skin-to-skin contact (Finigan & Davies 2004) or wrap in a warm towel for mother to hold

Third-stage management

See Figures 6 and 7.
(i) usually controlled cord traction (CCT) or modified Brandt–Andrews
(ii) physiological at mother's informed request
(iii) Brandt–Andrews method (rarely used now)
• Perineum/vagina/cervix examined to assess any trauma
• Placenta/membranes checked for completeness (see **Placental examination**)
• Blood loss estimated
• Routine observations – vital signs

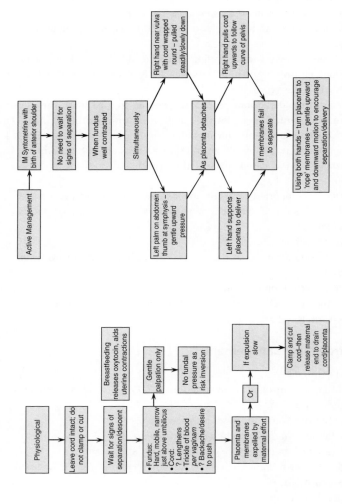

Figure 6 Management of third stage of labour – physiological and active.

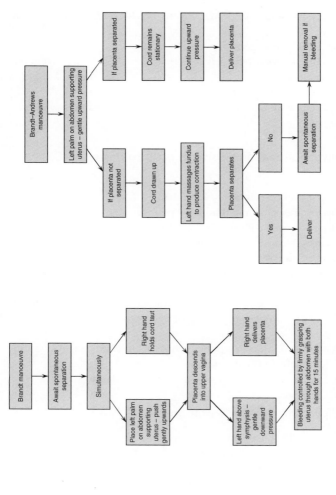

Figure 7 Management of third stage of labour – alternative active management.

- Uterus palpated to ensure good contraction
- Make mother comfortable
- Baby's top-to-toe examination (with mother) if satisfactory condition
- Apply ID bands in hospital setting (see **Identification of newborn**)
- Baby put to the breast prn
- Mother, partner, baby left for private time together (if condition allows)
- Contemporaneous records completed
- After approximately 1 hour, mother/baby transferred to postnatal area

Delivery of head in persistent occipito-posterior (OP) position

Face-to-pubes (see Figures 8, 9 and 10).
- Occurs after short rotation in OP position
- Head is usually deflexed – wider engaging diameter
- Increased risk of perineal trauma/? episiotomy
- Consider squatting position – increases diameters of pelvic outlet
- All-fours/kneeling position ? relieves backache associated with OP position
- Sinciput leading part; flexion of the fetal head is encouraged by exerting pressure with the fingers of the left hand towards the symphysis
- When the occiput sweeps the perineum the head extended slightly to release baby's glabella and face
- Remainder of the delivery conducted as previously

Delivery of a face presentation

See Figures 11, 12 and 13.
- May be primary presentation or, more commonly, secondary
- Associated with OP position – wider diameter delayed at pelvic brim, head completely extends, becoming mento-anterior position

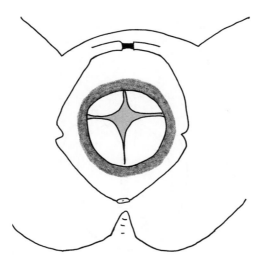

Figure 8 Persistent occipito-posterior position – landmarks on vaginal examination: anterior fontanelle, sagital suture, parietal bones.

- (NB: mento-posterior position will not deliver vaginally; insufficient pelvic space for occiput anteriorly)
- VEs kept to a minimum/performed very carefully during the first stage of labour – preventing tissues damage
- Considerable pressure to face from pelvic floor during descent through the birth canal – ? tissues damage – bruised/oedematous (inform woman/partner)
- Paediatrician present at the delivery – ? problems with resuscitation

Action

- Episiotomy necessary to prevent perineal trauma
- Maintain gentle pressure on sinciput, allowing mentum to deliver first under pubic arch
- Sinciput, vertex, occiput delivered by flexion

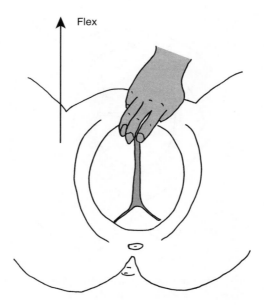

Figure 9 Persistent occipito-posterior position – delivery of the occiput: flex the head towards the symphysis pubis if deflexed as this allows the smaller diameter to come through the introitus. Allow the occiput to sweep the perineum.

- Avoid facial trauma whilst feeling round the neck for cord
- Continue as normal delivery; pass baby to paediatrician for examination/resuscitation
- NB: baby may have head retraction for a few days following delivery – ? severe bruising causing feeding problems/re-absorption jaundice – ? observe/manage in NNU

Student activity

Revise mechanisms of labour.

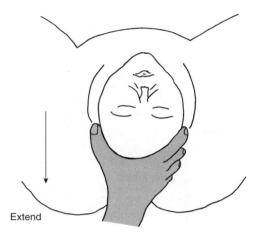

Figure 10 Persistent occipito-posterior position – delivery of the chin: when the occiput has been delivered, extend the head to bring the face under the sub-pubic arch and allow the chin to escape.

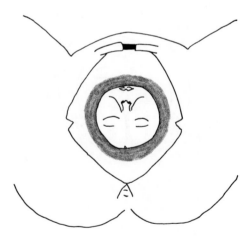

Figure 11 Face presentation – landmarks on vaginal examination: orbital ridges, nose, cheek bones, mouth.

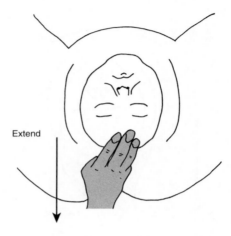

Figure 12 Face presentation – delivery of the chin: extend the head further to allow delivery of the chin from under the pubic arch.

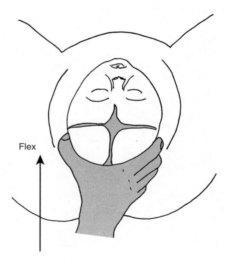

Figure 13 Face presentation – delivery of the occiput: when the chin is released, flex the head to allow the occiput to sweep the perineum.

Diabetes mellitus

- *Type I diabetes*:
  - ○ Pancreatic function is poor/non-existent
  - ○ Daily insulin by subcutaneous injection is required
  - ○ More common in younger people
- *Type II diabetes*:
  - ○ Some pancreatic function remains
  - ○ Oral medications either stimulate insulin production or aid glucose utilisation
  - ○ Onset commoner in older people
- *Impaired glucose tolerance (latent diabetes)*:
  - ○ Insulin adequate but glucose metabolism inefficient
  - ○ Occurs only at times of stress
  - ○ May develop into frank diabetes in later life
- *Gestational diabetes*:
  - ○ Occurs only during pregnancy (2–5% pregnancies)
  - ○ Resolves following childbirth
  - ○ May develop into frank diabetes in later life

Aetiology – gestational diabetes

- Remains uncertain; often unrecognised
- Generally presents in the third trimester
- Linked to raised placental hormones
- May be due to:
  - (i) inadequate insulin production for increased needs
  - (ii) abnormal carbohydrate metabolism
  - (iii) insulin resistance
- Women at greatest risk:
  - (i) ethnic groups
  - (ii) older women
  - (iii) family history of diabetes
  - (iv) previous history of gestational diabetes
  - (v) previous large baby
  - (vi) previous unexplained stillbirth/neonatal death
  - (vii) BMI >30

Diagnosis

- NICE (2008d) *Clinical Guideline 63* suggests that oral glucose tolerance test (OGTT) is the best way of diagnosing the condition
- Some units prefer fasting blood glucose levels >6.7 mmol/l or random blood glucose >7.8 mmol/l (laboratory test) – then OGTT
- OGTT: 75 g oral glucose given and blood taken 2 hours later:
  - (i) blood glucose levels >8 mmol/l = gestational diabetes
  - (ii) blood glucose levels 6–8 mmol/l = impaired glucose tolerance

Diabetes and pregnancy

Pre-conception

- Sub-fertility if poor control
- Identify severity of diabetic changes, i.e. nephropathy, neuropathy, retinopathy (kidney, nerve, eye)
- Discuss risks of worsening of complications; ? avoid pregnancy (informed choice)
- Treat complications
- 'Tight' control of blood glucose levels (5–6 mmol/l) improves pregnancy outcome
- Target range for HbA1c below 6.1% reduces risks of congenital malformations. If HbA1c is above 10%, should not contemplate pregnancy (NICE 2008d)
- Women offered monthly HbA1c assessment
- Women with Type 1 diabetes should be offered ketone testing strips and advised to test for ketonuria if hyperglycaemic or feeling unwell
- Type 1 diabetics may change over to insulin pump – may give better control
- Type II diabetics – change over to insulin multi-dose regime
- Care from diabetes specialist consultant and nurse
- Dietary advice from dietitian; includes folic acid 5 mg daily

Pregnancy

- Insulin requirements increase from 20 weeks
- Insulin dose/frequency may need changing
- Diabetic complications, especially retinopathy, may worsen
- Hypoglycaemic attacks may increase with 'tight' control
- Continue 'tight' control on blood glucose levels (5.5–6.0 mmol/l fasting) by dietary control and exercise
- Insulin – but hypoglycaemic attacks more likely and glucagon IM provided and partner/family instructed when and how to administer
- Increase blood glucose monitoring (urinary glucose unreliable)
- Strategies for coping with morning sickness
- Close liaison with diabetes specialists throughout pregnancy
- Early recognition/treatment of retinopathy
- Women should be reassured that if they maintain good control of blood glucose levels, the outcome for them and their babies is the same as for any other woman

Gestational diabetes

- Rapid specialist referral if suspected/diagnosed
- Dietary advice/weight reduction
- Insulin regime as indicated

Pregnancy and diabetes

Increased risk of complications, particularly when control is poor.

Maternal

- Infection
    - (i) UTI
    - (ii) vulvo-vaginitis, especially *Monilia* (thrush)
    - (iii) amnionitis which may lead to premature rupture of membranes
    - (iv) puerperal sepsis

- Cardiovascular
    (i) PPH risk (if polyhydramnios)
    (ii) PIH, pre-eclampsia, eclampsia risk
    (iii) proteinuria and oedema likely
    (iv) thromboembolic disorders risk
- Genital tract trauma due to large baby, with possible long-term consequences

Baby

- Miscarriage
    (i) spontaneous/induced
    (ii) higher incidence often linked to fetal abnormalities
- Preterm delivery
    (i) induced
    (ii) spontaneous
    (iii) caesarean section
- Oligohydramnios/polyhydramnios – associated with
    (i) large baby
    (ii) large placenta
    (iii) preterm labour
    (iv) congenital abnormalities:
        - cardiovascular
        - renal
        - central nervous system, e.g. anencephaly
        - caudal regression syndrome, i.e. sacral ageneses and lower-limb hypoplasia
        - skeletal
        - hypospadias (urethral opening on underside of penis)
- IUD – increased risk in last 3–4 weeks – associated with
    (i) high maternal glycosylated haemoglobin (HbA1c) reducing O_2 transfer across placenta
    (ii) maternal ketoacidosis
    (iii) maternal infection
    (iv) hypertensive disorders
- IUGR – due to
    (i) poor uterine perfusion/placental insufficiency
    (ii) fetal malformations

    (iii) maternal infection

    (iv) maternal hypertensive disorders

- Fetal distress in labour – due to

    (i) placental insufficiency

    (ii) maternal ketoacidosis

    (iii) prolonged labour

    (iv) shoulder dystocia

- Macrosomia, i.e. baby >4000 g (diabetic cherub) – risk of

    (i) perinatal/neonatal death

    (ii) prolonged labour

    (iii) shoulder dystocia

    (iv) birth injury

    (v) birth asphyxia

    (vi) instrumental/operative delivery

- RDS (SDS) (neonatal) – due to

    (i) high fetal insulin inhibiting surfactant production

    (ii) prematurity

- Hypoglycaemia (neonatal); blood glucose level <2.5 mmol/l (or lower – controversial); occurs $1-1\frac{1}{2}$ hours later, caused by fetal hyperinsulinaemia

- Polycythaemia (excess RBC), hyperviscosity (sticky blood) due to high maternal glycosylated haemoglobin (HbA1c) reducing O_2 transfer across placenta causing:

    (i) plethora (redness)

    (ii) cardiovascular disorders and tachycardia

    (iii) tachypnoea (rapid breathing) and respiratory distress

    (iv) convulsions

- Hypocalcaemia (low calcium) – 2–3 days after birth

    (i) increased muscle tone; twitching; convulsions

    (ii) associated with respiratory distress; asphyxia; acidosis

- Jaundice – 2–3 days after birth, due to:

    (i) increased haemolysis of RBC (polycythaemia)

    (ii) inhibited liver enzymes

    (iii) prematurity

- Infection – more prone

- Long-term outcome
    - (i) higher incidence of obesity
    - (ii) increased incidence of diabetes

Management – pregnancy

- Multi-professional team approach, ideally combined appointments
- Early antenatal booking
- Obstetric consultant to lead care
- ? Some community-based midwife care (depending on condition)
- Discuss plan of care with woman
- Regular ultrasound scans/biophysical profiles
- Date of pregnancy
- Identify abnormalities
- Retinal assessment offered in early pregnancy if not done in the previous year. If retinal assessment normal, repeat at 28 weeks; if abnormal repeat 16–20 weeks
- Monitor fetal well-being
- Blood monitoring:
    - (i) glycosylated haemoglobin (HbA1c) – venous blood
    - (ii) reagent strip with a meter at home – peripheral blood
- Early recognition/management of PIH/pre-eclampsia
- Early recognition/treatment of infections, especially UTI
- Hospitalisation for complications
- ? Estimation of fetal lung maturity 37–38 weeks (rarely amniocentesis/LS ratio)
- Consider optimal delivery time; NICE (2008d) recommends induction or C/S at 38 weeks
- Consider appropriate labour management; give women choice if possible

Management – labour

- Senior obstetrician, anaesthetist, diabetes specialist involved
- Experienced midwife supervising
- Usual labour management – vigilant for complications
- Follow labour guidelines of the unit for diabetes care

- Analgesia prn – ? epidural beneficial
- Clear fluids only orally
- IVI 10% glucose/dextrose at 10 g per hour (i.e. 100 ml per hour) – less fluid overload than 5% glucose
- IV insulin (using pump) according to blood glucose levels
- Peripheral blood glucose levels hourly using a reagent strip and meter
- Urinalysis for ketones
- ? Continuous electronic monitoring
- ? Fetal blood sampling; early identification of fetal compromise
- Preterm labour; maternal IM corticosteroids (observe for hyperglycaemia and ketoacidosis)
- Paediatrician at delivery
- Neonatal unit on standby
- Emergency caesarean section if in doubt about vaginal delivery

Management – postnatal

- Insulin requirements fall rapidly after delivery
    (i) halve insulin infusion immediately after third stage
    (ii) return to pre-pregnant insulin as soon as normal diet is taken
- Blood glucose monitoring continues
- Urinary glucose levels more reliable
- Prophylactic antibiotics following caesarean section
- Breastfeeding encouraged (increased carbohydrate without insulin increase)
- 6-week postnatal appointment
- Referral to diabetes clinic for follow-up
- OGTT at 3 months for gestational diabetics/advise long-term follow-up (risk of late-onset diabetes)
- Preconception advice prior to subsequent pregnancy
- Contraception – ? IUCD (infection risk), oral, barrier methods

Management – neonate

- Inform/support parents
- Baby with mother unless special care needed

- Remain in hospital until 24 hours old and maintaining blood glucose levels (NICE 2008d)

Hypoglycaemia

- Monitor blood glucose (see **Heel prick**)
  (i) HemoCue™ system (more accurate for low levels of glucose than reagent strip and meter)
  (ii) ideally, true blood glucose (TBG) on venous blood
- Early feeding
- Neonatal unit if symptomatic; IVI glucose

RDS (SDS)

- Neonatal unit
- Surfactant administered

Polycythaemia and hyperviscosity

- Early clamping of cord to prevent excess blood transfer
- NNU if symptomatic
- Exchange blood-for-plasma transfusion

Hypocalcaemia

- Monitor blood levels
- IM or IV calcium

Jaundice

Usual management.

Infection

Early recognition and treatment.

SGA/prematurity

Usual management.

Abnormalities

• Individualised management
• Echocardiogram if signs of heart murmur or abnormality (NICE 2008d)

Student activity

• Revise anatomy and physiology of the pancreas
• Revise signs, symptoms and diagnosis of diabetes
• Familiarise yourself with all types of insulin/administration
• Note your local policy and procedures for:
    (i) screening for gestational diabetes
    (ii) care of the diabetic woman during pregnancy, labour and puerperium
    (iii) neonatal care
• Further reading: Feig and Palda (2002); Glueck *et al.* (2002); *Clinical Guideline 63 – Diabetes in Pregnancy* (NICE 2008d); Platt *et al.* (2002)

Disseminated intravascular coagulation (coagulopathy) (DIC)

Disseminated, throughout the body; intravascular, within the blood vessels; coagulation, clotting.

Aetiology

• A syndrome (secondary to primary event)
• Widespread clot formation causes abnormal fibrinogen and clotting factor consumption; clotting mechanism fails – haemorrhage occurs

Primary event

• Severe tissue damage
• APH/PPH
• Amniotic fluid embolism
• Severe pre-eclampsia/eclampsia
• Prolonged IUD (intrauterine death)

- Septicaemia
- Inherited coagulation disorder
- Low platelets

Prevention

- Prevent, treat, manage primary event
- Coagulation defect screening/abnormalities aggressively managed

Management – initial

See Figure 14.

Management – subsequent

Postnatal debriefing and psychological support.

Complications

- Maternal death
- Sheehan's syndrome
- Renal failure
- Infection risk increased
- Psychological morbidity, e.g. post-traumatic stress (see **Postnatal depression**)

Student activity

- Note your local policy/procedures for DIC
- Familiarise yourself with intensive care charts/records/EWS/MEWS/ MOEWS (see Section 1)
- Further reading: Levi (2009)

Down's syndrome

- A genetic abnormality of chromosome 21, either trisomy (i.e. 3 instead of 2 chromosomes) or a translocation of a piece of one of the chromosomes on to another
- See **Antenatal screening**

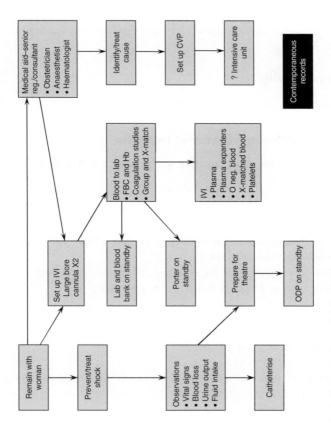

Figure 14 Disseminated intravascular coagulation (DIC).

• Down's Syndrome Association – offers information and support to parents and professionals
Langdown Down Centre,
2a Langdown Park,
Teddington, TW 11 9PS.
Tel: 0845 230 0372 Fax: 0845 230 0373
Email: info@downs-syndrome.org.uk http://www.downs-syndrome.org.uk

Student activity

Further reading: Skotko (2002); Tolliss (1995).

Drug-addicted mother and neonate

See **Substance-abusing mother and baby** and **Smoking in pregnancy**.

Eclampsia

See also **Pregnancy-induced hypertension (PIH) and Pre-eclampsia** and **MAGPIE trial**.

Fitting (like major epileptic fits) associated with childbearing – during pregnancy, labour or first 48 hours postnatally.

Signs and symptoms

• ? Evidence of pre-eclampsia/PIH
• Mother may 'feel strange'
• Premonitory stage – eyes may roll, mild facial and/or hand tremors
• Tonic stage – spasmodic muscle activity up to 30 seconds
  (i) clenched teeth/fists
  (ii) respirations stop = cyanosis
• Clonic stage – jerky/violent muscle movements may last 2 minutes
  (i) frothy saliva
  (ii) may bite tongue
  (iii) may inhale mucus/vomit
• Coma; deep unconsciousness; lasts minutes/hours; cyanosis fades

Management

See Figure 15.

Prevention

• Early and prompt treatment of pre-eclampsia (see **MAGPIE trial;** Neilson 2007)
• End the pregnancy – ? caesarean section

Consequences

• Status eclampticus, i.e. continual fitting – increased risk of:
• Maternal/infant morbidity
• Maternal death
  ◦ five cases between 1997 and 1999 (Lewis 2001)
  ◦ six cases between 2000 and 2002 (Lewis 2004)
  ◦ seven cases between 2003–2005 (Lewis 2007)
• Perinatal death (intrauterine hypoxia)

Student activity

• Compare/contrast eclampsia/epileptic seizure
• Further reading: Draycott *et al.* (2000); Duley *et al.* (2003); Sibai (2004a, 2004b, 2005)

Embolism

A moved clot of blood that commonly lodges in the lung (pulmonary – PE) or in the brain (cerebral), frequently having arisen from a DVT.

Cerebral embolism

Signs and symptoms

• Sudden collapse/death/unconsciousness
• Severe headache/pain
• Signs of cerebrovascular accident (CVA – stroke), e.g.
  (i) paralysis (limb, facial)
  (ii) dysphasia (difficulty speaking)

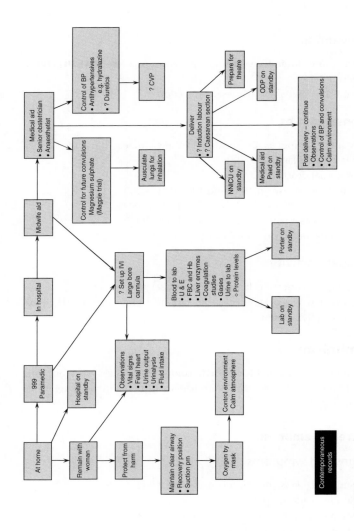

Figure 15 Eclampsia.

Diagnosis

- History
- CAT scan confirms

Pulmonary embolism

Signs and symptoms

Mild	*Severe*
Slight pyrexia	Obvious pyrexia
Slight dyspnoea (difficulty breathing)	Severe dyspnoea; coughing
Slight transient chest pain	Severe chest pain
Raised respiration rate	Cyanosis
Unproductive cough	Haemoptysis (coughing up blood)
	Respiratory arrest
	Death

Diagnosis

- History
- Chest X-ray/scan

Management

- Resuscitation prn
- Medical aid – obstetric team, physicians, anaesthetists
- Anticoagulants
- IVI
- Psychological support – mother, partner, family

Complications

- Death – thromboembolism is the commonest cause of maternal mortality in the United Kingdom (Lewis 2007)
- Long-term morbidity from respiratory damage (pulmonary embolism)
- Long-term morbidity from paralysis (cerebral embolism)
- Psychological morbidity
- Psycho-social effects on family

Student activity

Further reading: Drife (2007); Lewis (2007).

Epigastric pain

Pain in the upper abdomen/lower chest behind sternum.

Aetiology

- Heartburn, dyspepsia (indigestion), wind (see **Heartburn**)
- Oesophagitis (inflamed oesophagus due to acid reflux)
- Bleeding under liver capsule in severe (fulminating) pre-eclampsia, often before eclampsia

Management

- Differential diagnosis vital
- Indigestion, wind, oesophagitis – antacids
- Pre-eclampsia/eclampsia (see **Eclampsia** and **Pregnancy-induced hypertension/Pre-eclampsia**)

Epilepsy

Abnormal brain electrical impulses.

Types

Clinical seizure type and EEG findings denote classification, but is not always clear-cut.
- *Generalised seizures may*
  - be convulsive/not
  - involve jerking muscle movements (myoclonic)
  - involve body/limbs stiffening (tonic)
  - involve sudden tone loss, causing slumping/collapse (atonic)

- be severe (grand mal) tonic to clonic phase, with subsequent unconsciousness, possible cyanosis, incontinence, confusion and drowsiness on regaining consciousness
- involve sudden, brief altered consciousness (absence seizures/ petit mal)
- involve a stop in motor activity and then immediate recovery without confusion/any awareness of attack
- *Partial seizures possibly*
  - simple or complex
  - complex often arise in the temporal lobe (temporal lobe epilepsy)
  - consciousness altered
  - unilateral muscle jerking
  - speech affected
  - sensory hallucinations, e.g. smell, taste, flashing lights, hearing
  - memory/perception disorders, e.g.
    - (i) *déjà-vu*
    - (ii) objects appear large or small
    - (iii) feelings of unreality
  - dream state
  - strong emotional feelings, e.g. rage, fear, pleasure, displeasure
  - confusion and automated, repetitive behaviour, e.g. chewing, gesturing, walking in circles
- *Status epilepticus* – repeated major seizures without return to consciousness

Management

- Depends on type and frequency of seizures
- Common drugs used – carbamazepine (Tegretol), phenobarbitone, phenytoin (Epanutin), sodium valporate (Epilim)

Student activity

Further reading: additional information http://www.epilepsy.com/; http://www.epilepsyfoundation.org/

Epilepsy and pregnancy

- *Increased congenital abnormalities* (if treated/not) (screening of-fered), e.g.
    - congenital heart disease/defect (phenytoin)
    - cleft lip/palate (phenobarbitone)
    - NTD (carbamazepine, phenytoin, valporate)
- *Maternal/neonatal coagulation defects* (phenobarbitone)
    - IM vitamin K to mother during pregnancy/labour or if any bleeding
    - IM vitamin K to neonate

Pre-conception

- Neurological specialist advice regarding medication control
- Folic acid supplements – 5 mg daily
- Inform mother of potential risks

During pregnancy/postnatal

- Dangers of not treating outweigh treatment as seizures may
    - (i) increase/decrease/not change
    - (ii) re-occur after years without episodes
    - (iii) present for the first time
    - (iv) return to pre-pregnant state postnatally
- Breastfeeding suitable with most medications
- Risk of maternal death – 11 died during 2003–2005 (Lewis 2007)

Student activity

- Compare/contrast epileptic seizures and eclampsia
- Note your local policy for managing status epilepticus
- Further reading: Barrett and Richens (2002)

Episiotomy

See also **Perineal repair**.

Part of the midwife's role after perineal infiltration with local anaesthetic – mediolateral episiotomy in United Kingdom – avoiding trauma to Bartholin's glands/anal sphincter.

Aim

Enlarge vaginal introitus, facilitating safe delivery for mother/
baby.

Preparation

- Carefully explain procedure prior to labour/discuss likelihood during labour
- Seek informed consent (NMC 2008)
- Trolley with needles, syringes, local anaesthetic (lignocaine [lidocaine] 0.5% 10 ml or 1% 5 ml)
- Episiotomy scissors
- Maintain woman's dignity

Action

Anaesthetic

- Local anaesthetic drawn up into syringe
- Woman in semi-recumbent position; perineum swabbed/antiseptic solution
- Two fingers inserted into vagina; perineum lifted off fetal head
- Needle inserted beneath skin, 4–5 cm along line proposed for incision
- Piston of syringe withdrawn to ensure no blood
- Lignocaine injected as needle slowly withdrawn, about one-third of syringe contents
- Redirect needle before fully withdrawn; make two further injections on either side of original line; Fan-shaped area infiltrated.

NB: infiltration timing important to allow anaesthesia (unnecessary infiltration better than performing episiotomy without)

Incision

- Ideally performed during a contraction when perineum is thin/ distended
- Place two fingers into the vagina – to protect fetal head
- Open scissors, place blades along the line of infiltration

- Incision made during a contraction – a single deliberate cut the length of the blades
- Scissors removed/replaced on trolley
- Delivery of head follows almost immediately with next contraction – be prepared
- Continue as normal delivery
- NB: PPH possible from episiotomy; check blood loss

Erb's palsy (paralysis)

Arm weakness/paralysis in neonate due to damaged brachial plexus (nerve group in the lower neck).

Signs

Arm hangs loosely/palm turned backwards.

Aetiology

Neck stretching during breech/difficult delivery.

Management

- Information/explanation to parents
- Physiotherapy aids resolution
- Support for parents and further information from the Erb's Palsy Group: http://www.erbspalsygroup.co.uk

Exchange transfusion

Aims

- Removal of unconjugated bilirubin, antibodies and damaged cells
- Correct anaemia

Prior procedures if baby at risk

- Paediatrician at birth
- Immediate cord clamping/cutting – 5 cm stump left

- Cord blood – group, Hb, bilirubin, Coombs test (see Section 1)
- Hb < 12 g/dl with cord bilirubin >85 µmol/l (normal 5–16 µmol/l) – immediate exchange
- Hb > 14 g/dl with bilirubin <50 µmol/dl – treat as physiological jaundice
- Hb < 14 g/dl with bilirubin <50 µmol/dl – exchange 4–6 hours

Preparation

- Baby in NNICU
- Parents informed/supported
- Blood glucose, potassium, calcium – before and during
- Hb, bilirubin, blood gases, U & E before
- Maintain thermal environment
- Ensure clock with second-hand is available
- Resuscitation/monitoring equipment
- ? Vitamin K prior
- Quieten baby – ? dummy (sedatives may mask shock)
- Equipment:
  - (i) umbilical catheter
  - (ii) extension tube and 3-way tap
  - (iii) container for waste blood
  - (iv) calcium gluconate
  - (v) infusion stand and blood warmer
  - (vi) record chart

Action

- Senior paediatrician/sterile procedure approximately 2 hours
- Assisting midwife/nurse
- Fresh Rhesus-negative, ABO-compatible blood exchanged; 170–180 ml/kg (3 kg baby = 540 ml); calcium gluconate if stored blood used to counteract citrate (anticoagulant)
- Immobilise baby in splint
- Stomach empty – ? give dummy
- Procedure ? repeated 2–3 times

Umbilical vein technique

• Umbilical vein catheter passed; blood withdrawal/donation using 3-way tap
• About 5–20 ml blood is withdrawn and discarded
• Tap is turned, then equal amount of donor blood replaced ? blood warmer used

Two-site technique

• Peripheral artery/umbilical artery for withdrawal
• Peripheral vein for donation
• About 5–20 ml blood is withdrawn and discarded; simultaneous replacement with equal amount of donor blood via syringe pump/blood warmer
• Observations:
    (i) strict fluid balance/exchange
    (ii) vital signs – ? continuous ECG
    (iii) ? pulse oximetry
    (iv) general condition – colour, muscle tone

Post-transfusion care

• Umbilical vein/artery sutured or ligated prn
• Continue observations
• ? Phototherapy
• Repeat blood tests
• Baby not fed for 2–3 hours
• Parental information/support/care participation
• ? Oral iron later
• Paediatric follow-up

Dangers

• Over-transfusion
• Shock
• Necrotising enterocolitis (inflamed/ischaemic/obstructed bowel)

Student activity

Further reading: Maisels and Watchko (2003).

Face presentation

See also **Delivery technique**.
Head presenting fully flexed, occiput against shoulders.

Aetiology

- *Primary* – i.e. before labour, due to:
Abnormal fetus, e.g. anencephalic; fetal goitre (enlarged thyroid)
- *Secondary* – i.e. develops during labour, owing to:
  - extended brow presentation
  - oblique uterine position
  - lax uterine muscles
  - flat/abnormal pelvis
  - prematurity
  - polyhydramnios
  - multiple pregnancy

Diagnosis

- Abdominal palpation – difficult, possibly high presenting part
- VE (NB: avoid trauma from examination) (see Figure 11 for landmarks)
  - (i) ? high presenting part
  - (ii) orbital ridges/mouth felt (? sucked finger)
  - (iii) differentiate from anus of breech
  - (iv) oedema and bruising ? identification landmarks difficult

Management – pregnancy

- USS excludes abnormalities and multiple pregnancy
- ? X-ray pelvimetry excludes CPD

Management – labour

Usual care.

Management – delivery

See **Delivery technique**.

Fainting

Sudden loss of consciousness, full/partial.

Aetiology

- Not uncommon antenatally
- General/supine hypotension
- Anaemia
- Shock – physiological/emotional

Prevention

Avoid prolonged standing, supine position, sudden position changes, e.g. rapid rising from bed, very warm conditions (peripheral dilatation).

Management

- Recovery position
- Ensure clear airway
- Medical aid/ambulance if no rapid recovery/complications
- History to elicit possible cause
- Advice on prevention

Fetal distress

See also **Birth asphyxia**.

A compromised fetus due to acute/chronic lack of O_2 (hypoxia).

Aetiology

- Inadequate uterine circulation
- Placental insufficiency
- Cord occlusion
- Low maternal O_2
- APH
- Postmaturity
- Congenital abnormality
- Intrauterine infection
- Rhesus incompatibility
- Maternal shock – injury, haemorrhage due to:
  - (i) placental abruption
  - (ii) eclampsia
  - (iii) prolonged/precipitated labour
- Malpresentation, e.g. breech
- Cord compression – knot/prolapse
- Excessive sedation/analgesia
- Hypertonic uterine action
- Operative/instrumental delivery
- Shoulder dystocia

Associated factors

Sociological

- Low income, education
- Poor nutrition/general health
- Smoking/substance abuse
- Maternal age – >35, young teenagers

Maternal disease

- Hypertensive disorders (chronic or pregnancy-related)
- Cardiac, chronic renal, pulmonary
- Diabetes – poorly controlled
- Severe anaemia, haemoglobinopathies
- Epilepsy – poorly controlled

Signs – chronic

- Diminished fetal movements (FM)
- IUGR – noted on abdominal palpation
- USS/Doppler USS – diminished umbilical artery/uterine vessel flow
- Biophysical profile – diminished FM and breathing movements, oligohydramnios

Signs – acute and chronic

- Fetal heart auscultation – abnormalities in rate/regularity
- CTG
    - (i) reduced baseline variability
    - (ii) non-reactive pattern, i.e. no FH accelerations
    - (iii) severe bradycardia/tachycardia or reduced variability
    - (iv) late decelerations
    - (v) marked variable decelerations
    - (vi) sinusoidal pattern
- Meconium liquor – fresh from acute, old from earlier episode
- Fetal blood sample – pH at/below 7.20 (7.25 borderline)

Management – chronic

Antenatal

- Obstetric-led care
- ? Manage underlying cause
- Avoid strenuous exercise/work
- Regular monitoring of fetal well-being
- ? Preterm delivery

Labour

- Hospital birth
- Obstetric-led care
- Continuous CTG
- ? Instrumental/operative delivery
- Paediatrician at delivery
- ? NNICU on standby

Management – acute

- Medical aid – obstetric SHO/registrar
- Assess labour stage
- ? Fetal blood sampling
- ? Instrumental/operative delivery
- Paediatrician/midwife/nurse skilled in advanced resuscitation at delivery (see **Birth asphyxia**)
- ? NNICU on standby

Complications

- Intrauterine death (IUD)
- Perinatal/neonatal death
- Long-term morbidity:
  - (i) poor physical/intellectual development
  - (ii) cerebral palsy
- Parental and family stress/anxiety – long-term psycho-social consequences

Student activity

- Familiarise yourself with normal/abnormal CTGs
- Note your local policy on calling medical aid in fetal distress
- Observe biophysical profiles
- Further reading: Modder (2009)

Fitting

See **Epilepsy; Eclampsia; Jittery (twitching) baby**.

Forceps delivery

See **Instrumental delivery**.

Frequency of micturition

Abnormal frequency in PU.

Aetiology

- Physiology of pregnancy, i.e. pressure from gravid uterus on bladder
- UTI – e.g. cystitis, pyelonephritis

Management

- History aids diagnosis
- Dip stick urinalysis
- MSSU for culture/sensitivity (C & S)

Fundal height estimation (antenatal)

Recommended by NICE (2008a) (but not an exact science).

Aim

- Locate the uterine fundus measuring distance to symphysis pubis
- Compare with previous recordings to estimate fetal growth

Preparation

- Ensure privacy
- Woman to empty bladder
- Woman lying as flat as is comfortable (avoid supine hypotension)
- Explain procedure/gain consent
- Tape measure available
- Wash hands

Action

- Standing on woman's right, using left hand palpate upper abdomen until fundus located – place ulnar border of hand here
- Place free end of tape on upper border of symphysis pubis – extend to left hand
- Note measurement in centimetres
- Advise woman of findings, e.g. 30 cm – 30 weeks gestation
- Record in notes/chart on growth curve
- Deviation from normal – inform doctor

Fundal height estimation (postnatal)

- Controversial – ? discontinued
- Tape measuring imprecise/unhelpful when making clinical judgements
- Uterine consistency/loss *per vaginam* more appropriate

Student activity

Further reading: Baston (2004b); McAllion (2004).

Haemoglobinopathies

- A group of hereditary globin (protein of haemoglobin) abnormalities
- Haemoglobin (Hb) – normal:
  - has four iron (haem) atoms and four protein (globin) chains – half genetically from each parent (see Figure 16)
  - 98% adult Hb – two alpha and two beta chains (HbA) (see Figure 17)
  - 2% adult Hb – two alpha and two delta chains (HbA2) (see Figure 18)
  - Fetal Hb = two alpha and two gamma chains (adult Hb by 6 months) (see Figure 19)

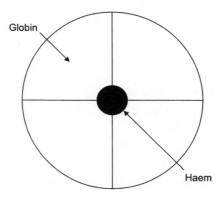

Figure 16 Haemoglobin composition: four iron (haem) atoms and four protein (globin) chains.

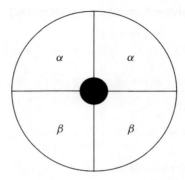

Figure 17 Normal adult haemoglobin HbA: 98% of adults – two alpha and two beta protein chains.

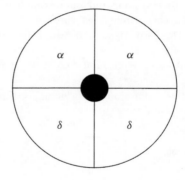

Figure 18 Normal adult haemoglobin HbA$_2$: 2% of adults – two alpha and two delta protein chains.

- Alpha chains – 141 amino acids (proteins or polypeptides) – each chain has two genes
- Beta, delta and gamma chains – 146 amino acids – each chain has one gene

General consequences of abnormal Hb

- Changes in O_2 affinity – cyanosis and polycythaemia (excess red cells)

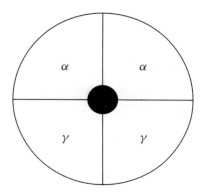

Figure 19 Normal fetal haemoglobin: two alpha and two gamma protein chains.

• Unstable molecules – excess haemolysis (breakdown) RBC – anaemia

Types of haemoglobinopathies

>300 – only two important in pregnancy.

Sickle cell condition (or sickle cell anaemia)

• Mainly West Africans, West Indians – less often Indians, Greeks, Cypriots
• Beta chain is affected – labelled HbS or HbC, depending on abnormality
• Inherited from one parent – HbAS or HbAC (heterozygous) – sickle cell trait (Figure 20)
• Inherited from both parents – HbSS or HbCC or HbSC (homozygous) – sickle cell disease (Figure 21)
• Sickle crisis may occur (see below)
  Consequences of HbSS or HbSC (HbCC no sickling occurs).
• RBC haemolysis may occur 17 days after cell production instead of the normal 120 days
• Anaemia/possibly jaundice from excess haemolysis

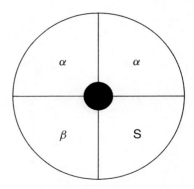

Figure 20 Abnormal haemoglobin – sickle cell trait: two alpha protein chains, one beta protein chain, one sickle protein chain.

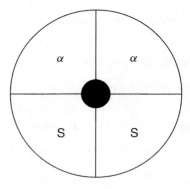

Figure 21 Abnormal haemoglobin – sickle cell disease: two alpha protein chains, two sickle protein chains.

- RBC sickle – (sickle cell crisis if severe) leads to:
  (i) blocked vessels
  (ii) soft tissue inflammation, e.g. abdomen, lungs, joints, organs (esp. kidneys)
  (iii) hepatosplenomegaly (enlarged liver and spleen)
  (iv) stroke/death

- Causes of sickle crisis
  (i) sudden temperature change
  (ii) dehydration
  (iii) infection
  (iv) alcohol
  (v) emotional stress
- Management of a crisis
  (i) analgesia; hospitalisation if severe; hydration; prophylactic antibiotics
  (ii) ? O_2; heparin; blood transfusion/exchange transfusion

Management in pregnancy

- Early booking (see website below regarding national screening policies)
- Genetic counselling for couple (ideally pre-conception)
- Diagnose fetus – CVS; amniocentesis; fetal blood via fetoscopy
- Offer TOP if fetus affected
- Obstetric/haematologist care
- FBC, Hb
- Routine infection screening, e.g. MSSU
- ? Prophylactic antibiotics, especially in labour
- Monitor fetal growth/well-being
- Liver function tests
- ? Blood or exchange transfusion if Hb low
- Adequate hydration in labour
- ? O_2 especially if drowsy
- No IUCD postnatally (infection risk), or combined oral contraception – progesterone-only and barrier methods suitable

Thalassaemia

Worldwide, most common haemoglobinopathy – prevalent around Mediterranean area:
- Alpha thalassaemia – 6 forms – commoner in Asians/East Asians (China, Hong Kong, Singapore, Malaysia)

- Beta thalassaemia – 10 forms – commoner in Greeks, Cypriots, Italians
- Gamma thalassaemia – affecting fetal haemoglobin

Consequences of thalassaemia

- Depends on type
- RBC haemolysis may occur 40 days after cell production (normally 120 days)
  - Alpha thalassaemia
    (i) alpha thalassaemia minor or trait (heterozygous) – one to two genes affected in one alpha protein (Figure 22) – asymptomatic
    (ii) three genes affected – two genes affected in one alpha protein and one in the other – very unstable – poor outcome
    (iii) alpha thalassaemia major (homozygous) – all four genes affected, i.e. two in each chain (Figure 23) – IUD or perinatal death (therefore no adults)
  - Beta thalassaemia: presents about 6 months after birth as adult Hb produced
    (i) beta thalassaemia minor (heterozygous) – gene in one chain affected (Figure 24)
      – Hb often low (10 g)
      – usually well
      – folic acid supplement – no iron unless deficient

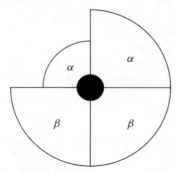

Figure 22 Abnormal haemoglobin – alpha thalassaemia minor or trait. One alpha protein chain affected (i.e. one or two genes).

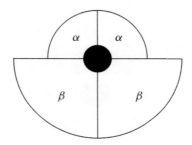

Figure 23 Abnormal haemoglobin – alpha thalassaemia major. Both alpha protein chains affected (i.e. all four genes).

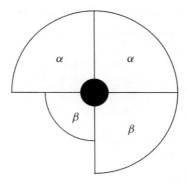

Figure 24 Abnormal haemoglobin – beta thalassaemia minor. One beta chain affected (i.e. one gene).

    (ii) beta thalassaemia major (homozygous) – each gene in both chains affected (Figure 25)
- hepatosplenomegaly (enlarged liver and spleen)
- bone deformities
- hypoxia and iron overload (due to haemolysis) – liver damage/ heart failure
- endocrine failure – growth retardation/restriction and gonad failure = infertility
- may survive until mid-adulthood if well managed

○ Gamma thalassaemia – IUD or perinatal death

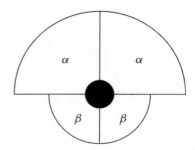

Figure 25 Abnormal haemoglobin – beta thalassaemia major. Both beta chains affected (i.e. both genes).

Management in pregnancy (thalassaemia minor)

• Early booking (see website in the following text *regarding* national screening policies)
• Genetic counselling for couple (ideally pre-conception)
• Diagnose fetus – CVS; amniocentesis; fetal blood via fetoscopy
• Offer TOP if fetus affected
• Obstetric and haematological care
• FBC and Hb
• Folic acid only, unless iron-deficient
• Infection screening

Student activity

• Diagrammatically depict inheritance as in PKU (see **Phenylke-tonuria [PKU]**), but substituting HbAA, HbAS, HbSS, HbSC
• Note your local policies regarding routine antenatal screening for haemoglobinopathies
• Further reading: National screening policy, Online: http://www.kcl-phs.org.uk/haemscreening/newborn.htm; Sickle Cell Society, Online: http://sct.sicklecellsociety.org

Haemorrhagic disease (Vitamin-K-deficient bleeding – VKDB)

Uncommon, potentially life-threatening bleeding due to lack of vitamin K 1–7 days after birth (commonly 3rd–4th day) or later.

Aetiology

Liver unable to synthesise clotting factors II (prothrombin); VII; IX; X owing to lack of vitamin K.

Contributory factors

- Prematurity
- Breastfeeding (human milk is low in vitamin K)
- Slow colonisation of normal gut flora (needed for vitamin K synthesis), e.g. due to delayed or prolonged feeding or antibiotics
- Perinatal hypoxia, birth asphyxia, trauma
- Oral anticoagulants antenatally
- Maternal anticonvulsants for epilepsy, e.g. phenobarbitone, phenytoin
- Neonatal liver disease (late-onset bleeding)

Signs

- Lethargic
- Pale
- Irritable
- Abnormal coagulation studies
- Abnormal bleeding:
    - (i) from nose, mouth
    - (ii) haematemesis (vomiting blood)
    - (iii) melaena (blood in faeces)
    - (iv) from skin and mucous membrane
    - (v) after heel prick
    - (vi) large cephalhaematoma
    - (vii) brain – seen on scan

Prevention

- Avoid oral anticoagulants antenatally
- Alternative anticonvulsants
- Prevent prematurity/perinatal compromise
- Establish early feeding

- Avoid prolonged antibiotics
- Routine prophylactic vitamin K with parental consent

NB: controversy *regarding* administration route, i.e. oral/IM.

Management

- Depends on severity
- Blood for coagulation studies; FBC; Hb; group and cross-match
- Special/intensive care
- Administration/repeat vitamin K
- Fresh frozen plasma
- Blood transfusion
- Information/support for parents

Complications

- Anaemia
- Neurological damage from cerebral haemorrhage
- Death

Student activity

- Note your local policy on vitamin K administration
- Further reading: Bushell *et al.* (2007); Hey (2003)

Haemorrhoids

Varicose veins in the rectum or anal area.

Aetiology

- Pre-existing prior to pregnancy/childbirth
- Chronic condition due to childbearing
- Pressure from the gravid uterus
- Progesterone relaxing smooth muscle of veins
- Straining during second-stage labour
- Obesity
- Constipation

Management

- Avoid forced pushing during second stage
- Prevent constipation: high-fibre diet, mild laxatives, e.g. lactulose
- Topical cream/ointment prn, e.g. Anusol
- Pelvic floor exercises
- Medical aid if severe

Student activity

Further reading: Quijano and Abalos (2005).

Headaches

Aetiology

- Not uncommon antenatally/postnatally
- Stress/fatigue
- Hypertension, especially fulminating pre-eclampsia
- Drug-induced, e.g. labetalol (hypotensive)
- Epidural anaesthetic – controversial if uncomplicated – known in dural puncture
- Severe pyrexia

Signs and symptoms

- Severe headache, ? associated visual disturbance, e.g. 'flashing lights'
- Headache – postural (not lying down); after dural puncture

Management

- History aids diagnosis
- Record BP
- Medical aid prn
- Specific management for cause

Heartburn

See also **Epigastric pain**.

Painful, burning sensation behind sternum, +/− simultaneous acid in the throat.

Aetiology

- Gastric acid reflux due to cardiac sphincter (oesophagus/stomach junction) relaxation (progesterone relaxes smooth muscle) – oesophagitis may develop
- Increased abdominal pressure from gravid uterus
- Specific food/drink

Management

- Advise small frequent meals, note 'trigger' foods
- Avoid very fatty, spicy, acid meals
- Drink between, instead of with, meals
- Avoid smoking/alcohol
- Avoid drinking at bedtime
- Lay propped-up in bed
- Antacids
- ? Complementary therapies
- Medical aid if simple remedies fail

NB: differential diagnosis of epigastric pain – see **Pregnancy-induced hypertension (PIH) and Pre-eclampsia** and **Eclampsia**.

Student activity

Further reading: Dowswell and Neilson (2009).

Heel prick – peripheral blood sampling

See **Neonatal screening**.

Aim – sampling

Early detection/management of:
(i) PKU
(ii) hypothyroidism

(iii) haemoglobinopathies, e.g. sickle cell disease
(iv) cystic fibrosis
(v) hypoglycaemia (blood glucose estimation), e.g. at birth, 2, 6, 12 hours prn
(vi) other tests, e.g. SBR, Hb

Aim – procedure

- Obtain peripheral blood for testing
- Prevent undue trauma to baby's heel (see Figure 26)
- Keep accurate records

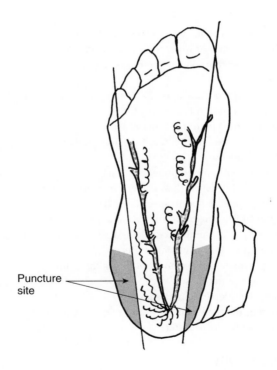

Puncture site

Figure 26 Foot with sites for heel prick.

Preparation

- Mother informed, consent obtained – may find it upsetting if baby cries
- Check baby's identity – complete record card
- Accurate completion of appropriate forms
- Baby comfortable/warm – especially heels
- Lancet, Steret or water, cotton wool, plaster
- Gloves worn (prevention of HIV/hepatitis B transmission)
- Baby held securely/lies in cot

Action

- Access heel
- Massage area of foot – encourages blood flow
- Swab heel – Steret or water for 30 seconds – allow to dry completely
- Automatic newborn lancet pierces skin, obtaining large blood drop
- For PKU:
    (i) place drop in circle of card – ensure soaked through
    (ii) repeat until four circles filled
    If capillary tube used (for other tests):
    (iii) ensure adequate blood in tube and tilt to mix
    For blood glucose:
    (iv) testing equipment for neonates, e.g. HemoCue™ system (more accurate for low levels than reagent strip and meter)
    (v) blood squeezed on to special device
    (vi) placed into the machine/read at appropriate time
    (vii) levels < 2.2 mmol/l considered significant (controversial) – ? lower without producing any signs
- Apply pressure with cotton wool to stop bleeding
- Plaster over puncture site
- Comfort baby/give to mother
- Document in records/advise mother *regarding* results
- Appropriately record results

Student activity

Further reading: Naughten (2005); UKNSPC (2008).

High vaginal swab (HVS)/speculum examination

- An intimate procedure – ? causing discomfort
- ? Midwife's/doctor's role
- HVS commonly taken when persistent/offensive vaginal discharge – using a speculum avoids contamination from the vulva/lower vagina
- Cusco's speculum commonly used – after insertion two blades opened, separating vaginal walls
- Speculum examination necessary to view the cervix:
  (i) in vaginal bleeding
  (ii) for diagnostic techniques, e.g. fibronectin detection, indicating premature labour
  (iii) for cervical screening

Aim

- Insert a speculum with minimum discomfort
- View the cervix/upper vagina
- Take HVS for detection of organisms
- Use other diagnostic swabs prn

Preparation

- Explain procedure/gain consent
- Dressing trolley with:
  (i) sterile speculum, gauze swabs, sanitary towel
  (ii) disposable gloves, cleansing fluid, ? obstetric cream/lubricant (? contaminates)
  (iii) swabs/culture medium prn
- Good light source
- Ensure privacy
- Ask woman to empty bladder
- Woman placed in dorsal position, knees flexed, thighs abducted

Action

- Wash hands/apply disposable gloves
- Vulva swabbed

- Speculum ? lubricated/gently inserted into vagina in upward/backward direction
- Open blades enabling viewing vagina/cervix
- Insert swab/sweep round upper vagina/cervix to obtain specimen
- Transfer to appropriate container/culture medium
- Remove speculum carefully to avoid pinching vaginal walls
- Dry vulva/position sanitary pad prn
- Make woman comfortable
- Explain result availability
- Maintain accurate records

History taking

- Full details:
  - medical
  - social
  - obstetric
  - present pregnancy
- History taken prior to:
- 'booking' a hospital bed for birth/midwife for home birth
  - Points to consider:

    (i) ? 'nerve racking' experience – particularly alone/in unfamiliar surroundings – may be better to book at home

    (ii) women carry their own notes

    (iii) Explanation of terminology and why certain questions are asked aids a woman's understanding

    (iv) adhere to request that confidential information, e.g. TOP, not be written in notes

Aim

NB: mothers may have difficulty remembering when faced with a barrage of questions.

(i) history taking is more than form filling

(ii) identify risk factors by taking accurate history

(iii) form the foundations of a trusting relationship

(iv) offer advice/information prn

(v) facilitate two-way discussion regarding care plans

Preparation

- Introduce yourself/other people present
- Ask what name woman/partner prefer to be called
- Put woman/partner at ease – explain procedure
- Work through history sheet – explain prn
- Use open-ended questions, e.g. 'How are you feeling?' rather than 'Do you have morning sickness?'
- Write clearly/legibly – check accuracy of recorded responses
- Give discussion time, particularly over issues of family history, e.g. genetic disease/familial problems
- Discuss whether referral to other agencies required
- Provide appropriate leaflets, e.g. on healthy eating, alcohol and smoking risks (oral information may be forgotten)
- ? Informally discuss preliminary care plans
- Discuss other things that may arise
- Give forms/information regarding blood tests, following physical examination
- Ensure relevant telephone numbers are documented

Student activity

- Familiarise yourself with your unit's history sheet/computer systems
- List routine blood tests at the first visit

HOOP (Hands On Or Poised) Study

A randomised controlled trial conducted during December 1994–1996 comparing perineal pain 10 days after two methods of conducting a normal delivery.

Method 1	Midwife's hands put pressure and flexion on the baby's head, i.e. to guard the perineum, with use of lateral flexion to deliver the shoulders
Method 2	Midwife's hands were poised and prepared to prevent rapid expulsion of the head, but otherwise did not touch the perineum or shoulders

Results

Women felt significantly less pain with Method 1, although the episiotomy rate was lower in Method 2.

Student activity

Further reading: McCandlish (1999, 2001).

Hyperemesis gravidarum

See **Nausea and vomiting**.

Hypoglycaemia – neonatal

See also **Heel prick**.

Definition

Levels <2.2 mmol/l considered significant (controversial) – ? lower without producing any signs.

Aetiology

Commoner after birth than at any other time of life, e.g. due to:
(i) Birth asphyxia
(ii) Prematurity
(iii) Starvation – see **Intrauterine growth restriction (IUGR)**
(iv) Sepsis – see **Infection – maternal; Infection – neonatal**
(v) Hypothermia
(vi) Transient hyperinsulinaemia – see **Hypoglycaemia (neonatal)** under **Diabetes mellitus**
(vii) Maternal IVI dextrose in labour
(viii) Rhesus incompatibility
(ix) Congenital heart disease
(x) Inborn errors of metabolism
(xi) Glycogen storage disease
(xii) Glucose-6-phosphatase deficiency
(xiii) Galactosaemia

Management

- Medical aid – paediatrician
- NNICU if severe
- Treat underlying cause if possible, e.g. infection
- Early oral feeding if well enough

Student activity

Check unit guidelines for neonatal hypoglycaemia.

Hypothermia – neonatal

Thermoregulation

- Heat loss due to:
    - (i) large surface area relative to body weight
    - (ii) large head relative to body
    - (iii) inability to shiver (muscle activity creates heat)
    - (iv) conduction – direct contact
    - (v) convection – air-cooled
    - (vi) radiation – heat given off
    - (vii) evaporation – drying moisture
- Heat maintenance aided by:
    - (i) drying baby
    - (ii) warm room/overhead heater/incubator
    - (iii) mother–infant body contact
    - (iv) wrapping in warmed bedding
    - (v) metabolism of brown fat (around kidneys, at back of neck, between shoulder blades) by noradrenaline (released after cold stimulates skin nerve endings)

Risk factors

- Preterm
    - (i) little/no brown/subcutaneous fat
    - (ii) immature thermoregulation centre
    - (iii) low glycogen stores

- Small for gestational age
    (i) little/no brown/subcutaneous fat
    (ii) low glycogen stores
- Birth asphyxia/prolonged resuscitation – acidosis; cold O_2; exposure
- Open lesions, e.g. exomphalus, spina bifida – heat loss
- Hypoglycaemia – reduced energy for metabolism
- Respiratory distress – altered metabolism/temperature control
- Sepsis – altered metabolism/temperature control
- Cerebral haemorrhage – shock; altered metabolism/temperature control

Complications

- Metabolic acidosis
- Respiratory distress/RDS (SDS)
- Apnoea
- Hypoglycaemia
- Death

Hypothyroidism

See **Heel prick** and **Neonatal screening**.
- Congenital (CHT) – cretinism
- Acquired – myxoedema

Identification of newborn at birth

Aim

- Accurately identify the newborn
- Ensure baby is given to correct parent(s)
- Parent(s)/witness(es) identification

Preparation

- Two identity bands with:
    (i) maternal surname, maternal/baby case note number
    (ii) infant's first name, date/time of birth
- Ask mother/partner to check details whilst in labour ward

Action

• Promptly after birth, securely attach band to baby's ankle(s)/wrist in presence of parent(s); ensure bands are not too tight/loose
• Document details in case records
• ? Write cot card with same information plus sex/weight
• Two midwives check bands if an unaccompanied woman has had a GA
• On receiving at the ward identity bands checked/records signed
• If one band becomes detached midwife informed; details checked again with mother; new band applied
• If both bands detached – two midwives check all babies before reapplying identity bands to the unnamed baby

Student activity

Identify your local protocol.

Incontinence

Involuntary passage of urine/faeces – frequent, intermittent, during stress, e.g. coughing, sneezing, laughing – ? retention with overflow.

Aetiology

• Pressure from gravid uterus
• UTI
• Bladder damage, especially to bladder neck, during labour/delivery or pelvic floor damage (nerves, muscle, connective tissue) – large baby; instrumental delivery
• Poor muscle tone, including anal sphincter
• Fistulae between vagina and bladder (vesico-vaginal) or vagina and rectum (recto-vaginal)

Management

• Prevention/early treatment of UTI
• Ensure bladder emptied after PU

- Prevent constipation
- Avoid pelvic floor trauma, e.g. instrumental delivery/prolonged second stage
- Early trauma detection/treatment
- Indwelling urinary catheter if severe trauma
- Pelvic floor exercises antenatally/postnatally – especially beneficial when large baby/instrumental delivery (Hay-Smith *et al.* 2008)

Student activity

- Learn/practice pelvic floor exercises – learn how to teach women/ implement in your care
- Further reading: Hay-Smith *et al.* (2008); Wesnes *et al.* (2007)

Induction of labour – alternative and 'natural'

Alternative methods have been used to stimulate the uterus, possibly in the hope of increasing circulating oxytocin/prostaglandins.

Women should be advised that effectiveness is unsupported by evidence; some may just cause significant discomfort; others, if under-taken, should be in strict privacy, usually at home!

Method examples

- Enemas
- Oral castor oil
- Hot baths
- Herbal remedies
- Acupuncture
- Nipple stimulation
- Clitoral stimulation
- Sexual intercourse (prostaglandins are high in seminal fluid so in theory may stimulate cervix)

Induction of labour – medical: uncomplicated pregnancy

See also **Augmentation/acceleration of labour**.

Indications

- Postmaturity – 41^{+0} to 42^{+0} weeks
- Hypertensive disorders
- Medical conditions – renal/heart disease, diabetes
- PROM
- Placental abruption (not requiring emergency caesarean section)
- Previous obstetric history, e.g. stillbirth
- Unstable lie (once corrected) (see **Transverse/oblique lie**)
- Rhesus isoimmunisation
- IUD
- Severe congenital abnormality
- Maternal request (controversial)

Contraindications

- Maternal objection
- Major CPD
- Suspected macrosomia
- Transverse/oblique lie
- Severe IUGR/fetal compromise
- Placenta praevia
- Severe APH
- Risk of unattended/rapid birth

Cautious use

- Minor CPD
- Multigravidas
- IUGR
- Mild/moderate IUGR/fetal compromise
- Uterine scar

Methods

See NICE (2008c).

All procedures with woman's informed consent (see Dimond 2006).

1. *Membrane sweep* – offered to:

    (i) Nulliparous women at 40 weeks

    (ii) All women at 41 weeks

    Procedure:

    Vaginal examination is performed; finger enters cervix to sweep the lower uterine segment to detach the membranes – may cause woman considerable discomfort; some bleeding and irregular contractions may result.

2. *Prostaglandin* (PGE$_2$) vaginal tablet/gel

    (i) postmaturity

    (ii) preterm rupture of membranes

    Procedure:

    ? Midwife's role in uncomplicated cases following medical discussion (see *The Code*: NMC (2008); *Midwives' Rules and Standards*: NMC (2004); *Standards for Medicines Management*: NMC (2007)).

    – Ensure placenta not low lying

    – Inform woman of risk of hyperstimulation

    – Induce in the morning if possible

    – PGE$_2$ for one cycle (maximum two doses) – one initial dose followed by second 6 hours later if not in established labour

    – Vaginal gel/tablets inserted into posterior fornix

    – Some women may wish to go home to await established labour – to contact midwife when contractions begin or no contractions by 6 hours

    – CTG when contractions begin to assess fetal well-being

    – Intermittent auscultation unless continuous CTG indicated (CTG should always be available)

    PGE$_2$ produces:

    – local cervical action/systemic uterine action

    – individual sensitivity:

    　　(i) ? rapid onset of strong painful contractions

    　　(ii) ? very rapid labour progression

    　　Methods 3 and 4 are only used for initial induction if PGE$_2$ unsuitable.

3. *ARM* (forewater amniotomy) (see also **Augmentation/acceleration of labour**)

4. *Syntocinon IV infusion* (see also **Augmentation/acceleration of labour**)

Induction of labour – IUD

Procedure

- Mifepristone (anti-progesterone) orally + vaginal PGE_2
- If previous C/S, reduced dose of prostaglandin

Student activity

- Revise physiology of labour
- Note your local policy and procedures
- Familiarise yourself with labour records
- Review the actions and doses of mifepristone and PGE_2
- Further reading: Boulvain *et al.* (2005); NICE (2008a, 2008c); NMC (2004, 2007, 2008)

Infection – maternal

Location

- Upper/lower genital tract
- Systemic, i.e. general
- Urinary tract
- Breast
- Coexisting, e.g. tonsillitis, appendicitis

Risk factors

See Lewis (2007):103.
- Obesity
- Impaired glucose tolerance/diabetes
- Impaired immunity
- Anaemia
- Vaginal discharge
- History of pelvic infection
- History of Group B streptococcal infection

- Amniocentesis and other invasive intrauterine procedures
- Cervical cerclage
- Prolonged SROM
- Vaginal trauma
- Caesarean section
- Wound haematoma
- Retained products of conception post miscarriage or post delivery

Associated factors

- Social disadvantage
- Poor nutrition, poor hygiene
- Poor general health
- Exposure to infection, e.g. STIs, contaminated food, cross-infection
- Stress/anxiety
- Prolonged/difficult labour

Types of organisms

- Bacteria
- Viruses
- Fungi
- Protozoa
- Spirochaete
- Parasites

Prevention

- Improve nutrition/hygiene, especially hand washing
- Pre-conception weight management in obesity
- Safe sexual practice (pregnancy = unprotected intercourse)
- Early identification/management of infection, especially UTI/genital tract
- Ensure bladder is emptied when PU
- Correct anaemia
- Maintenance of normal blood sugar levels in diabetes
- Avoid exposure to infections/microorganisms
- Effective labour management
- Prevent prolonged labour/dehydration

- Aseptic technique
- Minimal intervention, e.g. VEs/catheterisation
- Minimise trauma
- Prompt removal of retained products of conception
- Prophylactic antibiotics in 'risk' cases (see Ohlsson & Shah 2009)
- Avoid rough handling of breasts
- Correct fixing when breastfeeding

Complications

- Intrauterine infection – miscarriage; IUD; congenital abnormalities/infection
- Perinatal death
- Preterm labour/PROM
- Maternal morbidity:

    (i) physical – renal damage, scar tissue, secondary PPH

    (ii) psychological – fear of future pregnancies, resentment towards partner/baby

    (iii) psycho-sexual – loss of libido, dyspareunia (painful intercourse)

    (iv) social – unwilling/unable to fulfil normal social life
- Maternal mortality:

    18 direct and 16 indirect deaths from infection during 2003–2005 (Lewis 2007)

Management

- Depends on location of infection – early recognition and treatment essential
- Use of a MEOWS chart (see Section 1; Lewis 2007:247) aids early recognition

Student activity

- Review your local policies on recognition and management of infection during pregnancy, labour and postnatally – are MEOWS charts being used?
- Further reading: Fletcher and Ball (2006); Lewis (2007); NICE (2008a); National Clamydia Screening Programme Online: http://www.chlamydiascreening.nhs.uk

Infection – neonatal

Infection during the first 28 days of life:
- Early onset <5 days (average 20 hours)
- Late onset >5 days (average 20 days)

Neonatal defences

- Intact skin
- White blood cells inefficient, especially following hypothermia
- Immunoglobulins:
  (i) IgG – transplacental, i.e. passive immunity (low preterm)
  (ii) IgA – low levels (synthesised from 30 weeks gestation)
  (iii) IgM – low levels (present from 13 weeks gestation); increases following infection/oral feeding
  (iv) IgA – from colostrum and breast milk

High-risk factors

Maternal infection	General; intrauterine; vaginal; may be obvious infection or carrier e.g. group B *streptococcus* (GBS)
Membranes	Prolonged rupture; ARM; meconium-stained liquor; amnionitis
Monitoring labour	FSE; vaginal examinations
Labour	Prolonged; premature; difficult
Delivery	Difficult; operative
Compromised baby	Perinatal hypoxia; asphyxia; vigorous resuscitation; meconium aspiration; prematurity (low IgG levels); IUGR; multiple pregnancy; hypothermia; congenital abnormality; admission to neonatal unit – procedures; cross-infection

Routes of infection

Ascending vaginal flora	Anaerobic bacteria; *Streptococcus* (strep.) *pneumoniae*; *E. coli*; GBS

Transplacental	Rubella; *Listeria*; syphilis; gonorrhoea; *Varicella zoster* (chickenpox – a notifiable disease); HIV; toxoplasmosis
Intrapartum	Gonorrhoea; *Chlamydia*; *Herpes*; *Candida* (thrush)
Cross-infection	*Streptococcus epidermidis*; *Staphylococcus aureus*; haemolytic streptococcus; some viruses
Breastfeeding	HIV; yeasts

Signs and symptoms

General

- Pyrexia
- Hypothermia
- Temperature instability
- Weak cry
- Pallor
- Failure to thrive
- Jaundice
- Skin rash/pustules

Neurological

- Lethargy
- Irritability
- High-pitched cry
- Convulsions/jittery baby
- Hypotonia/hypertonia
- Neck rigidity
- Full fontanelle

Respiratory

- Tachypnoea/apnoea
- Intercostal recession

- Grunting
- Changes on X-ray

Cardiovascular

- Tachycardia/bradycardia
- Central cyanosis
- Anaemia
- Thrombocytopenia (low platelets)
- Abnormal white cell count

Gastrointestinal

- Poor feeding
- Abdominal distension
- Vomiting
- Diarrhoea
- Blood in stool (melaena)
- Enlarged liver/spleen

Diagnosis

- Signs and symptoms; history
- Early-onset recognition difficult
- First 24 hours only – gastric aspirate/external auditory canal (ear) swab
- Blood – culture; FBC; ESR and IgM (raised in infection)
- Culture – nose, throat, cord, rectal swabs; urine; endotracheal tube and IVI tips
- Lumbar puncture – culture CSF
- X-ray – chest; abdomen
- Ultrasound scan, e.g. brain

Management

- Depends on condition/severity – antibiotics/antiviral agents prn
- Medical aid (paediatrician or GP if mild late onset)
- May need to treat mother e.g. if gonorrhoea, *Chlamydia* or GBS identified

Complications

- General infection
- Skin infections
- Pyoderma (septic spots)
- Pemphigus neonatorum
- *Candida* (thrush – buttocks)
- Paronychia (nail bed)
- Mucous membrane – oral *Candida*
- Umbilical cord (risk of systemic spread)
- Septicaemia (growth of organisms in blood)
- Meningitis/encephalitis
- Respiratory distress/pneumonia
- UTI
- Gastro-enteritis
- Ophthalmia neonatorum (eye infection – especially gonorrhoea, *Chlamydia*)
- Necrotising enterocolitis (NEC) – inflamed necrotic bowel
- Convulsions
- Death
- Long-term neurological conditions

Student activity

- Consider antenatal advice on prevention
- Review local preventive practice during labour
- Elicit protocol for obtaining medical aid in the community
- Further reading: Fletcher and Ball (2006); Heath *et al.* (2009); Jones *et al.* (2009); Ohlsson and Shah (2009); Vergnano *et al.* (2005)

Initial newborn examination

- Part of midwife's role following delivery – mother/father present
- 'Top to toe' physical examination and auscultation of heart/ lungs – ? paediatric role or extended role of midwife
- (see also **Postnatal examination – baby**)

Aim

- Detection of abnormalities
- Record findings accurately in case notes
- Inform mother/father of findings
- Alert paediatrician prn

Preparation

- Explain procedure to parent(s) – invite observation
- Maintain baby's temperature (see **Hypothermia – neonatal**)

Action

- Assess Apgar score prior to examination
- Observe muscle tone/response to stimuli
- Listen to the cry/? colour changes
- Axillary temperature
- Two people weigh – inform parent(s)/record
- Measure length/head circumference prn
- Work from head to toe:

  (i) head – size, shape, symmetry of skull: feel suture lines/fontanelles

  (ii) face – ? two normal eyes, which both open

  (iii) nose – two patent nostrils

  (iv) lips/mouth – ? cleft lip/palate, teeth, 'tongue tie'

  (v) ? chin normally developed

  (vi) ? ears normal shape/structure, position on head (? in line with the eyebrows)

  (vii) neck – front/back ? abnormal swellings

  (viii) skin folds/pads of fat between shoulders

  (ix) arms – ? normal length compared to body, normal position/joints

  (x) hands – count digits; check for webbing/abnormal appendages; examine palmar creases

  (xi) chest – ? symmetrical; ? normal rib cage/diaphragm movement, normal nipples for gestation

(xii) abdomen – ? normal configuration/cord insertion; ? swellings/
abnormalities/gut/abnormal discharges

(xiii) genitalia – boys: ? urethral opening at tip of penis, normal
scrotum/descended testes; ? abnormal swellings

(xiv) genitalia – girls: ? normal labia – separate ? normal urethral/
vaginal openings

(xv) anus – ? normal situation/patency

(xvi) hips – test for dislocation/instability (see **Barlow's test** in
Section 1) – ? paediatric role

(xvii) legs – ? normal length compared to body/appearance/
position; ?normal knee joint

(xviii) feet – ? position; count digits; check for webbing/abnormal
appendages

(xix) back – run fingers along length ? abnormal indentations/
swellings/hair tufts

(xx) neural tube openings obvious

- Document findings in records (NMC 2009)

Student activity

Further reading: Williamson *et al.* (2005).

Insomnia

Inability to sleep.

Aetiology

- Physiological/psychological
- Discomfort of gravid uterus, especially in late pregnancy
- Minor disorders of pregnancy – heartburn, cramp, sciatica, carpal
tunnel syndrome, congested sinuses
- Frequency of micturition
- Anxiety/worry about pregnancy, baby, own health, sociological
factors
- Depression, ? early sign postnatally
- Bereavement

Management

- Depends on cause
- Change of position during pregnancy
- Investigate frequency of micturition
- Effective communication: enable the expression of concerns/anxieties
- Information prn
- Encourage family support/practical help
- Counselling prn
- Early identification/treatment of depression
- Alternative therapies, e.g. acupuncture, aromatherapy (with caution – expert advice), yoga, music/relaxation therapy

Instrumental delivery – Forceps delivery

- Speeds up delivery of fetal head – protects fetus/mother from undue trauma/exhaustion
- Not a midwife's role
- May be undertaken in theatre to enable rapid C/S if failed delivery

Prerequisites

- Cervix fully dilated
- Bladder empty
- Membranes ruptured
- Head engaged
- Denominator identified
- Effective uterine contractions
- Adequate anaesthesia – pudendal block, epidural, low spinal
- Episiotomy
- Informed consent

Aims

- Assist obstetrician
- Support woman/partner throughout
- Maintain contemporaneous records

Preparation

- Two midwives – assist obstetrician/receive baby
- Trolley prepared for normal delivery
- Sterile pack obstetric forceps – obstetrician determines type:
  (i) deep rotational, e.g. Kielland's
  (ii) mid-cavity delivery, e.g. Neville Barnes's, Haig Ferguson's, Simpson's
  (iii) low-cavity delivery, e.g. Wrigley's
- Urinary catheters – non-retaining and retaining
- Adequate needles, syringes, local anaesthetic, suture materials
- Inform paediatrician
- Effective resuscitation equipment

Action

- Place woman in lithotomy position, wedge under one side (prevents supine hypotension)
- Open forceps pack/required equipment, e.g. for infiltration/ pudendal nerve block
- Keep woman/partner informed of progress
- Advise woman *regarding* pushing prn
- Midwife receives baby as normal – shows to mother/passes to paediatrician (ID labels)
- Syntometrine given with birth of anterior shoulder unless contraindicated, e.g. in pre-eclampsia
- Syntocinon may be given
- Assist with perineal repair
- Remove legs from stirrups/make woman comfortable

Instrumental delivery – Ventouse delivery

May be part of midwife's extended role
- Speeds up delivery of fetal head
- ? Prevents caesarean section in late first-stage labour

Prerequisites

These are the same as for a forceps delivery but the cervix need not be fully dilated

Aims

As for forceps delivery.

Preparation

As for forceps delivery, but substitute sterile silastic cups, tubing, vacuum extractor (electronic or hand pump), metal chain and handle.

Action

- Presentation confirmed
- Silastic cup applied to fetal head as near to occiput as possible
- Vacuum applied slowly from $0.2\,\text{kg/cm}^2$ to $0.8\,\text{kg/cm}^2$
- Ensure cup is secure/apply steady downward traction as the mother pushes
- Head rotated if necessary
- Episiotomy prn
- Use steady gentle traction to follow the arc of the curve of Carus (see Section 1) through the pelvis and continue forward and upward as the head is born, i.e. continuing the curve
- Vacuum released and cup removed carefully
- Syntometrine given with birth of anterior shoulder unless contraindicated
- Continue as for forceps delivery

After birth

- Perform initial observations
- Maintain records accurately
- NB: increased complication risk for mother/baby ? observe longer in labour ward

- Discuss reasons for instrumental delivery with mother
- Advise mother that chignon (large bruised swelling) will subside after ventouse

Student activity

Further reading: NICE (2007).

Intrauterine death (IUD)

Fetal death. Expulsion of fetus – miscarriage at <24 weeks or stillbirth >24 weeks.

Aetiology

- Often unknown but there may be a history of previous fetal loss
- Chronic maternal causes:
  - (i) diabetes
  - (ii) cardiac, respiratory, renal disease
  - (iii) essential hypertension
  - (iv) smoking, substance abuse
  - (v) low socio-economic status
  - (vi) cholestasis
  - (vii) advanced maternal age
  - (viii) significantly high/low BMI
- Acute maternal causes:
  - (i) PIH/pre-eclampsia/eclampsia
  - (ii) systemic infection, e.g. toxoplasmosis; viral; bacterial
  - (iii) STIs, e.g. syphilis; herpes
  - (iv) intrauterine infections, e.g. viral; bacterial
- Placental causes:
  - (i) poor implantation
  - (ii) poor function – poor uterine blood flow, infarcts (small, old abruptions)
  - (iii) abruption
  - (iv) cord knot/entanglement/compression

- Fetal causes:
    - (i) congenital abnormality, e.g. cardiac
    - (ii) IUGR
    - (iii) postmaturity
    - (iv) malpresentation
    - (v) shoulder dystocia
    - (vi) Rhesus incompatibility
    - (vii) intrauterine infection
- Uterine causes:
    - (i) hypertonic uterine action
    - (ii) ruptured uterus
    - (iii) obstructed labour

Minimising risk

(i) well-balanced maternal diet

(ii) folic acid supplements (pre-conception and early pregnancy)

(iii) vitamin supplements prn

(iv) stop smoking/avoid passive smoking

(v) avoid infection/early recognition and management

(vi) avoid sudden illicit drug withdrawal

(vii) obstetric team management when 'at risk'

(viii) specialist liaison, e.g. physician prn

(ix) maternal information on recognition/rapid reporting of:
- complications, e.g. bleeding, infection
- abnormal/absent fetal movements

(x) effective monitoring of maternal/fetal well-being

(xi) early/prompt intervention prn

Signs

- Absent FM
- No FH auscultated with Pinard's stethoscope/Sonicaid
- No FH/FM on USS
- X-ray (not commonly used now):
    - (i) Spalding's sign (skull bones overlapping)
    - (ii) Robert's sign (gas in vessels/heart)

Management

Antenatal

- Sensitive information to mother/family
- Psychological support
- Informed choice about options:
  (i) await spontaneous abortion/labour
  (ii) generally hospital birth; if mother wishes home birth, inform supervisor of midwives
  (iii) induced abortion/labour
- Blood for FBC, Hb, clotting screening – weekly until delivered

Labour – known IUD

- Senior obstetric management
- Usual physical care
- Provide:
  (i) privacy/quiet room
  (ii) continuity of care/experienced midwife
  (iii) information/support to woman/family
- Neonatal resuscitation equipment/CTG monitor removed from room
- Cot remains
- Ensure up-to-date blood results, especially clotting profile
- Discuss analgesia*
- Discuss choices:
  (i) seeing/holding/bathing baby
  (ii) naming baby
  (iii) keepsake, e.g. lock of hair, hand/footprint, photograph of baby/family (if unwanted initially kept in case note and made available later)

---

*totally pain-free/heavily sedated labour experience may leave the mother with unreal feeling – unfulfilled meaningless experience/lack of achievement, almost negating pregnancy

    (iv) post-mortem examination

    (v) religious support/ceremony

    (vi) funeral/cremation – (hospital can arrange cremation)

- De-briefing/support for staff

Postnatal

- Information ? repeated, supported with written details
- Debriefing counselling
- Observe for postnatal depression
- Family support**
- ? Contraception/pre-conception advice
- Follow-up obstetric/paediatric appointment – 6 weeks
- ? Support agencies referral e.g. SANDS (see **Stillbirth and Neonatal Death Society**)
- GP/HV liaison
- Debriefing/support for staff

Long term

Possible consequences for mother, father, and family may include:

- Anxiety
- Deliberate social isolation
- Depression
- Post-traumatic stress
- Obsessive compulsive disorders
- Eating disorders
- Alcohol or substance abuse
- Relationship/family conflicts
- Reluctance for another pregnancy
- High anxiety during subsequent pregnancy

**inform family that leaving baby clothes/equipment ? helps the grieving process; ? prevents negation of pregnancy

Student activity

• Note your local policy and procedures
• Review the latest perinatal death statistics in CEMACH reports at the Centre for Maternal and Child Enquiries (CMACE) on http://www.cmace.org.uk
• Further reading: Brownlee and Oikonen (2004); Callister (2006); Schott and Henley (2007); Wallbank and Robertson (2008)

Intrauterine growth restriction (IUGR)

Aetiology

Often unknown – ? maternal/fetal.

Maternal risk factors

• Major organ disease – lungs, heart, kidney
• Hypertension – existing; pre-eclampsia; PIH
• Diabetes
• Significantly high/low BMI
• Poor nutrition – ? linked to social deprivation
• Smoking, drug, alcohol abuse
• Blood disorders – severe anaemia; sickle cell disease
• Epilepsy (poorly controlled)
• Severe infection

Fetal/placental risk factors

• Placental insufficiency after abruption
• Some congenital abnormalities, e.g. heart and renal
• Intrauterine infection – rubella, *Cytomegalovirus*, toxoplasmosis
• Rhesus incompatibility
• Cord compression e.g. entanglement

Management

- Early recognition
  (i) USS for serial growth measurements
  (ii) biophysical profile, noting fetal limb/body/breathing movements and tone
  (iii) amniotic fluid levels
  (iv) Doppler studies, noting umbilical artery blood flow
- Treat cause if possible, e.g. hypertension, anaemia
- Avoid prolonged pregnancy
- Delivery in consultant unit with NNICU (if transferring, accompanied by an experienced escort)
- ? Preterm delivery, induction of labour/caesarean section
- Careful monitoring during labour
- Paediatrician at delivery

Complications

- Intrauterine death
- Perinatal death
- Fetal distress in labour
- Birth asphyxia
- Meconium aspiration
- Those associated with SGA/prematurity (see **Small for gestational age**)

Student activity

Further reading: Miller *et al.* (2008).

Intravenous cannulation/infusion (IVI)

Insertion of IV cannula – ? midwife's role after correct training/ according to unit policy (not students' role).

NB: the following procedures provide only a basic overview to enable a student to assist with cannulation – further reading is advised to enhance knowledge.

Aim

- Establish venous access for IVI/bolus drug admistrations
- Prevent infection
- Keep accurate records

Preparation

- Dressing trolley/tray for aseptic technique
- Cannula (often a Venflon) – a thin plastic tube with needle inside – needle pierces the skin to enable the tube to be inserted into the vein – needle is removed once this is done
- Swabs, micropore tape, tourniquet, sharps box
- Transparent sterile dressing
- IVI fluid – ensure correct fluid; check expiry date
- Giving set – ensure correct type, especially if pump being used
- Pump/stand
- Close gate clamp on giving set and insert correct end into fluid bag using aseptic technique
- Run fluid through set ready for connecting to cannula – no air bubbles – ensure that end to link to cannula remains sterile
- Procedure explained/consent gained
- Choose site to minimise woman's discomfort – e.g. left arm if right-handed
- IVI chart

Action – insertion

- Disposable gloves worn
- Apply tourniquet
- Check for and palpate prominent veins
- Cleanse area
- Open cannula aseptically
- Ensure vein is stable using fingers of non-dominant hand
- Insert cannula into vein
- Ensure blood flow
- Giving set attached to cannula

- Cover/secure with transparent sterile dressing
- Record in records/IVI chart
- Check infusion site regularly ? swelling, redness, tenderness

Action – removal

- Close gate clamp on giving set
- Undo dressing/tape holding cannula in place
- Gauze swab over insertion area
- Apply pressure/remove cannula slowly
- Maintain pressure to stop bleeding/apply dressing
- Remove cannula from giving set – discard both safely
- Record date/time/any abnormalities, e.g. swelling

Student activity

- Observe 'running the giving set through' and practice under direct supervision initially to ensure you are able to safely undertake procedure, especially in an emergency
- Observe cannulation to enable you to assist midwife/doctor in procedure
- Check your local policy to ascertain if you are able to remove a cannula following training
- Further reading: Dougherty (2008a, 2008b); Ingram and Lavery (2007); Morris and Tay (2008); Scales (2008b)

Jaundice

Maternal – aetiology

- Severe hyperemesis gravidarum (pregnancy sickness)
- Hepatitis (liver inflammation) due to infection, often viral; or drugs
- Liver damage, e.g. due to severe pre-eclampsia/eclampsia; alcoholism
- Cholestasis, i.e. impaired liver function (see **Cholestasis**)
- Obstructed biliary tract

Management

- Urgent medical aid
- Treat underlying cause

Neonatal – aetiology

- Physiological jaundice:

    (i) common, in normal baby generally uncomplicated (exacerbated/serious if preterm)

    (ii) haemolysis (breakdown) of surplus erythrocytes (liver unable to cope with increased bilirubin) possibly due to late cord clamping (especially after Syntocinon – McDonald & Middleton 2008) or strong uterine contractions leading to increased blood volume

    (iii) breastfeeding – breast milk causes alteration of bilirubin metabolism

    (iv) haematoma – haemolysis of large haematoma/bruising increases bilirubin levels

    (v) drugs – e.g. diazepam (Valium); salicylates (aspirin)

- Haemolytic jaundice:

    (i) abnormal RBC breakdown – maternal antibodies from ABO or Rhesus incompatibility

- Infection:

    (i) intrauterine – rubella, toxoplasmosis, *Cytomegalovirus*

    (ii) neonatal – viruses, bacteria – UTI, cord infections, septicaemia

- Obstruction:

    (i) congenital biliary tract abnormalities

- Metabolic:

    ○ inborn errors of metabolism/enzyme disorders, e.g.

    (i) cystic fibrosis

    (ii) hypothyroidism

    (iii) galactosaemia

- Miscellaneous:

    ○ increased haemolysis due to:

    (i) large intake of maternal IVI glucose/IVI oxytocin

    (ii) traumatic birth

Prevention

• Avoid prematurity; birth trauma; excess IVI glucose/oxytocin; causative drugs
• Prompt cord clamping in active third stage of labour (balance with advantage of baby's increased Hb – McDonald & Middleton 2008)
• Early feeding minimises physiological jaundice
• Early recognition/management of blood incompatibilities (particularly if antibodies)
• Prevention of intrauterine/neonatal infections

Management

• Maternal history
  ◦ Blood group and antibodies
  ◦ Antenatal/intrapartum health
• Neonatal history
  ◦ Onset/depth of jaundice (in good light) – visual 'measure' of depth inaccurate (Keren *et al.* 2009)
  ◦ General condition – alertness, feeding, urine/stool colour, signs of infection
• Notify paediatrician if moderate/severe; symptomatic (see Activities of a midwife, *EU Second Midwifery Directive 80/155/EEC* in NMC (2004))
• Investigations
  ◦ Bilicheck (see Briscoe *et al.* 2002)
  ◦ Blood for SBR, FBC, Hb, group, antibodies, U & E
  ◦ Infection screening – culture urine, blood, swabs, ? CSF (lumbar puncture)
  ◦ Screening for metabolic disorders
• Admission to NNU prn
• Phototherapy/Biliwrap/Bilibed
• Drugs
  (i) phenobarbitone aids bilirubin metabolism – used cautiously (sedative effect ? inhibit feeding)
  (ii) oral iron to correct anaemia (caused by RBC haemolysis)
• Exchange transfusion
  In severe cases of haemolytic disease, sepsis or anaemia

- Parental care
  Information/support, encourage breastfeeding/participation in special care

Complications

- Anaemia
- Poor feeding
- Consequences of underlying cause of prematurity, infection
- Kernicterus (yellow staining of brain tissue)

Student activity

Further reading: Briscoe *et al.* (2002); Deken (2008); Keren *et al.* (2009); Truman (2006).

Jittery (twitching) baby

Small trembling limb movements, ? accompanying eye movements (convulsion more obvious).

Aetiology

Cerebral irritation.
(i) hypoxia
(ii) infection
(iii) jaundice
(iv) drug withdrawal
(v) metabolic disorders, e.g. hypoglycaemia, hypomagnesaemia, hypocalcaemia (low blood sugar, magnesium, calcium); hypernatraemia (high blood sodium)

Management

- Notify paediatrician (see Activities of a midwife, *EU Second Midwifery Directive 80/155/EEC* in NMC (2004))
- Identify cause
  (i) history
  (ii) observation

- Screening
  (i) infection
  (ii) blood – FBC, glucose, bilirubin, electrolytes, gases
- Anticonvulsants, e.g. phenobarbitone
- Treat cause
- Information/reassure parents

Complications

Convulsions – cerebral anoxia, brain damage, death.

Ketonuria

- Urine contains ketone bodies (acetone)
- Individual's breath may smell 'acidy sweet'
- May have central nervous system effects on mother/fetus

Aetiology

Fat metabolism due to lack of carbohydrate; waste product = acetone.

Cause

- Lack of insulin for carbohydrate metabolism, i.e. diabetes
- Inadequate carbohydrate intake, e.g. severe vomiting, starvation diet
- Excessive carbohydrate metabolism, e.g. prolonged labour
- Dehydration aggravates condition

Management

- Treat underlying cause appropriately
- Carbohydrate replacement, e.g. oral fluids/food; IVI glucose
- Urinalysis
- Fluid balance

Local Supervising Authority (LSA)

The 16 LSAs in the United Kingdom provide statutory midwifery supervision as required by the Government Act called the *Nursing and Midwifery Order 2001*, Statutory Instrument 2002 no. 253. They control the standard of midwifery services by advising service commissioners and providers and the standard of midwifery practitioners through midwifery supervision. All midwives (employed or independent) must have a designated supervisor of midwives (herself a practising midwife). Supervisors provide professional support and guidance; monitor individual and unit practices; have a disciplinary role in cases of alleged misconduct; and must ensure that midwives practise legally. Midwives must notify their intention to practise annually to their LSA via their supervisor in order to practise as a midwife.

Student activity

• Note references to LSA in your *Midwives' Rules and Standards* (NMC 2004)
• Identify your LSA and your local supervisors; discuss their duties
• Further reading: the LSA website Online: http://www.midwife.org.uk

MAGPIE trial

An international, randomised trial involving more than 80 hospitals in over 23 countries. Recruitment began in 1998, aiming to obtain 14,000 women. Coordinated in Oxford, the trial compared mortality and morbidity following IV treatment of pre-eclampsia. Clinical information was collected in hospital until postnatal discharge; at 3 months with a postal survey; and at 4 years at child follow-up.

Further reading: Duley and Watkins (1999).

Malpresentation – fetus

- A presentation other than vertex (NB: not malposition of the vertex)
- (see **Breech; face presentation;** and **Brow presentation** and **Transverse/oblique lie**)

Aetiology

Consider the following:
- Powers:
  - (i) uterine/abdominal muscles
- Passages:
  - (i) uterus – shape, liquor volume, structural anomalies
  - (ii) pelvic shape/size
- Passenger:
  - (i) fetal size/position
  - (ii) placental position

Maternity action

(NB: Maternity Alliance closed in 2005).

Established in 2008 – a national charity acting as advocates for pregnant women, their partners and children from pre-conception onwards.

Contact details:

Unit F5 89-93 Fonthill Rd,

London, N4 3JH.

Tel: 020 7281 7816

http://www.maternityaction.org.uk

Maternity benefits

- Free prescriptions in pregnancy and for 12 months post-delivery
- Free dental care in pregnancy and for 12 months post-delivery
- Free eye tests and podiatry in some cases
- Free milk, infant formula, fruit and vegetables for low-income families – Healthy Start Scheme

- Paid time off for antenatal care (proof of attendance required by employer)
- Paid time off for parent education if during work time

Monetary benefits

- Statutory maternity pay (SMP) or Contractual Maternity Pay if employer has own scheme
- Maternity allowance (MA)
- Incapacity benefit (ICA) – if not entitled to the others
- Statutory sick pay (SSP)
- Health in Pregnancy Grant
- Sure Start maternity grant (if on low income)
- Leave entitlement could include:
    (i) Maternity leave – ordinary and additional
    (ii) Paternity leave
    (iii) Parental leave
    (iv) Statutory adoption leave (SAL) and pay
    (v) Additional maternity leave (AML):
- Amount of benefit changes in April of each year
- Once child registered – child benefit may be claimed and Child Trust Fund initiated

Student activity

Further details: Department of Works and Pensions Online: http://www.dwp.gov.uk or government website on http://www.Direct.gov.uk

Maternity services liaison committees

Part of Care Service Improvement Partnership, the committees provide local forums for service users, providers and commissioners to meet to work together to ensure maternity services meet local needs. A website funded by the Department of Health: http://www.mslc.org.uk provides useful information.

Meconium liquor

See also **Fetal distress**.
- Meconium-stained liquor:
  - Fresh = thick, obvious stool
  - Old = passed during pregnancy, prolonged dark staining
- Quantifying the type and amount of meconium is inexact

Aetiology

- Fetal hypoxia – increased gut peristalsis and relaxation of anal sphincter
- Breech presentation
- Postmaturity

Management

Antenatal

(i) identify cause
(ii) monitor fetal well-being
(iii) ?? amnioinfusion with saline to dilute
(iv) ? deliver

Labour

(i) continuous CTG
(ii) close liquor observation
(iii) paediatrician, midwife, nurse skilled in advanced resuscitation at delivery

Neonate

(i) airway suction under direct vision, i.e. using laryngoscope/via ET tube to prevent inhalation – difficult to do when baby is actively gasping
(ii) O_2 – possibly via ventilator
(iii) homeostasis of blood gases

(iv) chest X-ray

(v) ECG

(vi) surfactant into respiratory tract

(vii) inhalation of nitric oxide

Complications

(i) Meconium aspiration:
  ○ *in utero* – fetal gasping movements
  ○ at birth – baby gasps, inhaling secretions in pharynx/trachea
(ii) Birth asphyxia
(iii) Respiratory distress/RDS (SDS)
(iv) Chemical pneumonitis (inflamed lungs)
(v) Pneumothorax – air into chest cavity, via damaged/collapsed alveoli
(vi) Perinatal/neonatal death
(vii) Long-term morbidity

Student activity

• Participate in simulated resuscitation of newborn
• Further reading: Lim and Arulkumaran (2008)

Medium chain acyl-CoA dehydrogenase deficiency (MCADD)

See **Heel prick** and **Neonatal screening**.

This enzyme deficiency is due to an inherited autosomal recessive gene affecting metabolism of medium-chain fatty acids.

Disorder characteristics

See UKNSPC (2007).

• Northern European white ethnic origin
• May not be clinically apparent at birth
• Symptoms may develop during infancy – occasionally asymptomatic during lifetime

- Inability to metabolise stored fat – unable to use energy reserves
- Build-up of medium-chain fatty acids
- Hypoglycaemia without ketones – especially in illness/fasting
- Seizures; brain damage; death in severe cases

Management

- Early detection and monitoring
- Avoid fasting – especially during illness

Mendelson's syndrome

Damaged respiratory tract from inhaled acidic vomit causing bronchial tree/alveoli spasm; resulting in scarring, respiratory distress, cyanosis and tachycardia.

Aetiology

Vomiting caused by:

(i) slow gastric emptying/lax cardiac sphincter (progesterone influence)

(ii) gravid uterus displacing stomach

(iii) possible side effect of pethidine/anaesthetic

Prevention

(NB: critical times – induction of anaesthesia/initial recovery).

- Routine nil by mouth prior to elective surgery
- Nil by mouth during normal labour has been much debated – NICE guidelines (2007) suggest women may drink (isotonic, i.e. sports drinks, may be beneficial) and have light diet unless opioid analgesia or risk factors for GA
- Routine administration oral antacid/ranitidine (Zantac) when risk of GA (NICE 2007)
- IM antiemetic with initial pethidine, e.g. prochlorperazine (Stemetil), metoclopramide (Maxolon)
- Vigilance during anaesthetic induction – Sellick's manoeuvre (cricoid pressure)

- Experienced obstetric anaesthetist
- Recovery position/careful observation post-operatively
- Readily available, effective suction equipment

Management

- Maintain respiratory function/blood gas levels
- Special care in an ICU, mechanical ventilation prn
- Prevent complications, e.g. respiratory infection
- Information/support for woman, family

Complications

- Long-term morbidity from damaged respiratory tract
- Mortality

Student activity

- Read and discuss your unit policy on eating and drinking in labour
- Further reading: Fraser and Mukhopadhyay (2009); NICE (2007)

Mid-stream specimen urine (MSSU)

Aim

To obtain uncontaminated specimen for laboratory testing – commonly culture and sensitivity (C & S)/ward testing.

Preparation

- Explain procedure
- Swabs for cleansing area
- Sterile container
- Correctly labelled laboratory forms

Action

- Instruct woman to wash genitalia
- Initial urine flow into toilet, catch mid-stream specimen into receiver/container

- Finish passing urine into toilet
- Appropriately labelled container/forms to laboratory prn
- Ward testing:
    (i) observe colour, odour, ? debris
    (ii) insert reagent strip/time according to manufacturer's instructions
    (iii) read results
- Record in notes

Multiple pregnancy/births

Simultaneous development of two/more embryos.

Incidence

Increased due to assisted fertility treatment.

Diagnosis

- Ultrasound (early pregnancy)
- Abdominal palpation:
    (i) uterus large for dates/many fetal parts felt (suspected)
    (ii) three poles (buttocks/head) identified
    (iii) two fetal hearts heard with difference >10 bpm

Pregnancy

Possibly normal

Complications

- Exaggerated minor disorders
- Increased fluid retention (increased hormones)
- Low-lying placenta (large placental site)
- Polyhydramnios
- Malpresentation
- Anaemia

- PIH/pre-eclampsia
- UTI

Management

Pregnancy

- Treat complications prn
- Discuss with mother – vaginal delivery/caesarean section prn
- Hospital birth advised – if mother's informed choice is home, notify supervisor of midwives

Labour

- First stage:
  (i) senior obstetrician's care
  (ii) depends on maternal condition, fetal lie/presentation
  (iii) ARM/Syntocinon with great caution prn
  (iv) usual labour care
  (v) sedatives/analgesia used cautiously (? small babies); epidural appropriate
  (vi) ? continuous electronic monitoring (twin machines available)
  (vii) prepare room for two babies, e.g. delivery pack/cots/resuscitation equipment
  (viii) obstetrician, paediatrician, anaesthetist, NNU on standby
- Second stage – anticipated vaginal delivery:
  (i) obstetrician/paediatrician present; midwife delivery/ies if cephalic
  (ii) *no* Syntometrine with first delivery
  (iii) identify first twin and placental end of cord (e.g. one cord clamp)
  (iv) palpate abdomen to confirm lie/presentation/FH
  (v) VE to confirm presentation/position/station
  (vi) ARM if suitable/uterus contracting – ? Syntocinon if not contracting
  (vii) vaginal delivery if cephalic/breech – caesarean section if complications

(viii) Syntometrine IM with second birth

(ix) identify second twin and placental end of cord (e.g. two cord clamps)

- Third stage:

    (i) as normal – beware of risk of PPH

    (ii) Syntocinon infusion continued for 1–2 hours

    (iii) placental examination as normal; note number of placentae as potential indicator of zygosity

- Postnatal:

    (i) physical/psychological/practical adjustment needed

    (ii) breastfeeding possible

    (iii) extra support from midwife initially prn

    (iv) family support at home prn – ? financial help/child care for higher multiples

    (v) ? support from voluntary organisations, e.g. TAMBA (see subsequent entry)

- Neonates:

    (i) remain with mother if conditions allow

    (ii) NNU if necessary

National Childbirth Trust (NCT)

A national charitable organisation based in London with local branches and members: a pressure group campaigning to improve maternity services, with some research being undertaken and educational activities via publications and study days. Volunteers offer information/support in pregnancy, childbirth and early parenthood: parent education classes (a fee usually required) and breastfeeding support (usually by phone but occasionally hospital/home visits). The organisation tries to make services, activities and membership fully accessible to everyone, enabling parents to make informed choices.

National Childbirth Trust,

Alexandra House, Oldham Terrace,

Acton, London, W3 6NH.

Tel: 0300 33 00 770 for enquiries

Tel: 0300 33 00 772 pregnany and birth line

Tel: 0300 33 00 773 early pregnancy line

Tel: 0300 33 00 771 breastfeeding line
http://www.nctpregnancyandbabycare.com

Nausea and vomiting

• A mild condition common in early pregnancy/primigravidas; possibly debilitating (although a 'minor disorder').
• Moderate/severe, i.e. hyperemesis gravidarum (hyper – excess; emesis – vomiting; gravidarum – related to pregnancy).

Signs and symptoms

Mild

• Commoner in the morning, particularly on waking; may last all day
• Food/drink aversions, e.g. tea, coffee, fatty foods
• Eating/drinking possible

Moderate/severe

• Continuous vomiting/no oral intake
• Signs of dehydration, i.e. dry mouth/skin; ketonuria; oliguria (poor/no urine output); halitosis (bad breath); sunken eyes
• Weight loss
• Exhaustion
• Drowsiness
• Disorientation

Aetiology

• Not always clear-cut
• Raised hormone levels, especially in early pregnancy
• Oestrogen and hCG (human chorionic gonadotrophin from placenta)
• Thyroid activity (severe cases)
• Reduced gastric motility with/without reflux oesophagitis
• Pre-eclampsia
• Multiple pregnancy

- Psychological factors, e.g. unwanted pregnancy (controversial)
- Fetal genetic abnormality
- Hydatidiform mole
- Incidental conditions, e.g. infection (especially UTI); gastro-enteritis; peptic ulcer; hiatus hernia

Management

Mild

- Individual trial-and-error solutions – no consensus of evidence on effectiveness
- Small, frequent, light meals, avoiding spicy and fatty foods (see Wills & Forster 2008)
- Dry toast/biscuit before rising and frequently during the day
- Soda water
- Vitamin B_6 (pyridoxine) – avoid overdose
- Ginger – biscuits, capsules, stem ginger
- Complementary therapies, e.g. acupressure (sea bands for travel sickness), acupuncture or hypnotherapy; homeopathy (see Dimond 2006; Rule 7, NMC 2004)

Moderate/severe

- Medical aid (Rule 6, NMC 2004)
- Admission to hospital
- History
- Observations – vital signs; fluid balance; urine output
- Investigations, e.g. urinalysis/MSSU; infection screening; USS; FBC, Hb, U & E;
- IVI – Hartmann's solution or dextrose/glucose; ? added potassium
- Antiemetic, e.g. prochlorperazine (Stemetil) or metaclopramide (Maxolon)
- Basic nursing care
- Oral fluids/light diet prn
- ? Termination of pregnancy if improvement fails/condition becomes life-threatening

Student activity

Further reading: Lacasse *et al*. (2009); McParlin *et al*. (2008); Wills and Forster (2008).

Neonatal screening

See **Heel prick, Hypothyroidism, Medium chain acyl-CoA dehydrogenase deficiency (MCADD), PKU**.

• A national programme – began in 1961 for PKU; 1981 for congenital hypothyroidism (CHT); 2004 for cystic fibrosis; 2009 for MCADD

• Over 60,000 screened annually in UK – >90% of babies

• Part of the midwife's role to obtain blood (with mother's informed consent) – ideally on fifth day after birth (day of birth counts as day 0)

Student activity

• Refer to *Standards and Guidelines for Newborn Blood Spot Screening*

• UK Newborn Screening Programme Centre Online: http:// newbornbloodspot.screening.nhs.uk

Neural tube defect (NTD)

A collective term for several central nervous system abnormalities, i.e.:

(i) anencephaly – absent skull vault/poor brain development (incompatible with life)

(ii) cerebral meningocele – involves the skull, commonly the posterior fontanelle

(iii) hydrocephalus – raised CSF causes large head

(iv) microcephaly – small skull vault, ? failed brain growth

(v) spina bifida – the spinal area

Aetiology

• Failed normal fetal growth

• Linked to lack of folic acid before conception/during early fetal development

• Microcephaly linked to intrauterine infection, e.g. rubella, toxoplas-mosis
• Genetic
• Drugs, e.g. rifampicin (for TB)

Recognition

• Antenatal screening – blood for AFP; amniocentesis; USS
• Initial neonatal examination
• Neonatal USS
• Hydrocephalus – wide, bulging fontanelles

Reduce risk of occurrence

• Avoid antenatal infection – rubella immunisation; effective hygiene, e.g. with cats
• Routine folic acid 4 µg (0.4 mg) (5 mg if high risk – NICE 2008b) 3 months pre-conception and first trimester
• Department of Health is considering mandatory fortification of bread or flour with folic acid (Food Standards Agency 2007)

Management

• Early antenatal detection ? offer TOP
• Neonatally depends on condition
• Paediatric referral
• Parental information/support

Complications

• Parental stress/anxiety, rejection
• Hydrocephalus – CPD, obstructed labour; caesarean section
• Increased infection risk
• Long-term morbidity – physical, psychological, social for parents/child

Student activity

Access the Food Standard Agency website http://www.food.gov.uk for up to date information on folic acid fortification.

Obesity in pregnancy

Body mass index (BMI) – method of assessing height–weight ratio to identify appropriateness of an individual's weight. Calculation – see Section 1. <20, underweight; 20–25, normal weight; >25, overweight; ≥30 at booking in pregnancy, obese – significant.

Risks

See Lewis (2007):26.

Increased risks for mother

- Maternal death or severe morbidity
- Cardiac disease
- Spontaneous first trimester and recurrent miscarriage
- Pre-eclampsia
- Gestational diabetes
- Thromboembolism
- Post-caesarean wound infection
- Infection from other causes
- Post-partum haemorrhage
- Low breastfeeding rates

Increased risks for baby

- Stillbirth and neonatal death
- Congenital abnormalities
- Prematurity

Management

- Pre-conception weight reduction is the ideal (see Barrowclough 2009) – obese women may have difficulty conceiving
- Inform woman of possible risks *tactfully* (most overweight people are sensitive about their weight/body image)
- Discuss diet, nutrition, exercise – avoid strict dieting – referral to dietician if needed

• Frequent weighing may be counterproductive and intimidating – no ideal weight gain in pregnancy – possibly about 8–10 kg – will be influenced by psycho-social and biological factors
• Monitor BP – large cuff may be needed
• Be alert for UTI and gestational diabetes
• Attendance at specialist (bariatric) clinic if available
• Care planning for risk reduction related to the list above

Student activity

• This is an increasingly important issue; therefore raise your awareness of the topic further
• Attend your local bariatric clinic if available
• Further reading: Barrowclough (2009); Cedergren (2007); Couch and Deckelbaum (2008); Crafter (2009); Heslehurst *et al.* (2007); Lewis (2007); National Research Council & Institute of Medicine (2007); NICE (2008a)

Occipito-posterior (OP) position

A malposition of the occiput which lies in the posterior of maternal pelvis towards a sacroiliac joint, either right (ROP) or left (LOP) or directly towards the sacrum (OP).

Aetiology

• Often unclear
• Pelvic shape, e.g. android, anthropoid, flat sacrum
• Pendulous abdomen
• Anterior placenta

Diagnosis

Pregnancy – alerting signs

• Abdomen appears flattened/slightly depressed below umbilicus
• Fetal limbs on both sides

- Back palpation difficult/impossible
- FH heard just below umbilicus/on flank
- Backache
- Failed/late engagement of fetal head – wide presenting part (if deflexed head)
- Prolonged discomfort under xiphisternum/breathlessness

Labour – alerting signs

- Abdominal examination
- Suprapubic/back pain, especially during contractions
- Excessively painful or poor contractions
- Delayed head descent/advancement
- Prolonged labour
- VE:
    (i) high presenting part
    (ii) cervix loosely applied, possibly oedematous
    (iii) slow, uneven cervical dilatation
    (iv) urge to push before cervix is fully dilated

Labour – confirming signs

VE:
(i) anterior fontanelle either central or anterior
(ii) posterior fontanelle possibly just tipped posterior
(see **Delivery technique** and Figure 8).

Mechanisms

Flexed head

- Lie longitudinal
- Vertex presenting, flexed attitude
- ROP or LOP position
- Suboccipito-frontal diameter (10 cm) engages
- As occiput reaches pelvic floor long rotation to OA occurs
- Normal delivery (see **Delivery technique** and Figures 9 and 10)

Deflexed head

- Lie longitudinal
- Vertex presenting
- Military attitude
- ROP/LOP
- Occipito-frontal diameter (11.5 cm) engages
- As descent takes place one of the following occurs:
  - (i) flexion occurs as above
  - (ii) partial extension occurs – brow presents (no vaginal delivery)
  - (iii) complete extension occurs – face presents
  - (iv) if deflexed attitude persists:
    - – sinciput reaches pelvic floor
    - – short rotation (45°) of sinciput to anterior, direct OP
    - – face to pubes delivery
    - Or
    - – occiput attempts long rotation to OA but
    - – becomes caught on prominent ischial spines – deep transverse arrest
    - – fetal head rotated using Kielland's forceps/Ventouse
    - – head delivery using mid-cavity forceps, e.g. Simpson's or Ventouse

Management – pregnancy

Anterior rotation of occiput/back *may* be helped by:
- periodically maintaining forward position, e.g. hands–knees, swimming
- lateral position for resting
- avoid prolonged, deep reclining position, e.g. on sofa, in bed, in car

Management – labour

- Close monitoring of progress
- Information, support, encouragement
- Leaning forward position/hands–knees position
- Back massage ? relieves pain
- Use bath/birthing pool, especially in hands–knees

- Maintain empty bladder
- Adequate analgesia – ? epidural
- Augmentation of labour prn
- Instrumental/operative delivery prn

Complications

- PROM (ill-fitting presenting part)
- Prolapsed cord (ill-fitting presenting part)
- Prolonged labour – first/second stage
- Difficulty/inability PU
- Premature pushing urge
- Trauma – cervix, perineum
- Instrumental/operative delivery
- Fetal hypoxia
- Excessive moulding of fetal skull
- Birth trauma
- Perinatal mortality
- Long-term morbidity for mother/child
- Psychological trauma/post-traumatic stress

Student activity

- Practice mechanisms with doll and pelvis
- Simulated VE with OP positions
- Further reading: Hunter *et al.* (2007)

Oligohydramnios

Definition

Reduced volume of amniotic fluid for gestation.

Aetiology

Poorly understood but occurs in:
- Placental insufficiency
- Post maturity >42 weeks – placental insufficiency

- Fetal abnormality e.g. Potter's syndrome – renal agenesis; therefore no fetal urine to contribute to liquor volume
- Preterm rupture of membranes (PROM) – liquor draining faster than production
- Maternal hypertensive conditions
- Twin-to-twin transfusion

Diagnosis

- Uterus small for dates
- Fetus feels compact
- USS – amniotic fluid index – poor sensitivity for diagnosis – pools of liquor 1–2 cm deep (no consensus on liquor amounts in the literature)

Potential complications

- Compression deformities e.g. face, talipes
- Fetal skin dry and leathery
- Hypoplastic lungs (poorly developed) – lack of liquor into lungs during fetal breathing movements
- IUGR
- Miscarriage
- Preterm birth
- Stillbirth

Management

- Information to mother
- USS for fetal anomalies
- Amnioinfusion (possibly serial) – infusion of IV fluids (normal saline commonly used) into amniotic sac (see NICE 2006) – risk of infection; will drain out if PROM
- Paediatrician at birth

Student activity

- Revise formation of liquor
- Visit ultrasound department to see amniotic fluid index measurement – elicit definition of oligohydramnios in your maternity unit

• Further reading: Crafter (2009); Magann *et al.* (2000); NICE (2006)

Ophthalmia neonatorum

Definition

Purulent discharge from the eyes of the newborn within 21 days of birth – may lead to corneal scarring/blindness if untreated.

Signs

• Yellowish discharge from eye, commonly at 3–4 days
• Inflamed/swollen eyelid
• ? Inflamed conjunctiva

Aetiology

• Infection, e.g. *E. coli*, *Staphylococcus*, *Streptococcus*, gonorrhoea (*Neisseria gonorrhoeae*), *Chlamydia trachomatis;* viral, e.g. *Herpes simplex* (rare) (occasionally none identified)
• Poor infection resistance, e.g. prematurity, traumatic birth
• Blocked tear ducts
• Maternal genital tract infection
• Cross-infection (including professionals!)
• Poor hygiene

Prevention

• Recognition/treatment of maternal infection
• Avoid contact with infected people
• Effective hygiene, especially hand washing
• Minimal routine eye cleansing

Management

• Notify paediatrician (see Activities of a midwife, *EU Second Midwifery Directive 80/155/EEC* cited in NMC (2004)).
• Eye swab culture/sensitivity

- Bathe eye with sterile water/cool boiled water at home – swab once inside to out (NB: hand washing!)
- Chloramphenicol eye drops/ointment – ? before swab results
- Tetracycline drops/ointment for *Chlamydia*
- ? Systemic antibiotics
- Mother and partner treated if gonorrhoea/*Chlamydia*

ORACLE trial

Overview of the role of antibiotics in curtailing preterm labour and early delivery. Begining in 1994, this international randomised controlled trial, funded by the Medical Research Council, aimed to see if treatment with broad-spectrum antibiotics would lessen neonatal mortality and morbidity due to PROM and preterm birth.

Student activity

- See **PROM, Preterm labour, Neonatal infections, Maternal infections**
- Further reading: Kenyon (1995); Kenyon and Taylor (2002); King and Flenady (2002)

Parent education

- Can be:
  - Formal/informal
  - Planned/opportunistic
  - Individual/group sessions
  - Antenatal, intrapartum, postpartum
  - At home, in a community/hospital setting
  - NHS or private, e.g. National Childbirth Trust (NCT)
- Before undertaking consider:
  - How people learn – active participation ('doing'/experiencing) aids learning
  - Why people learn – relevance to needs

- When people learn: self-initiated learning lasts longer
- Who learns:

   (i) mother, father, siblings, grandparents

   (ii) the community (see Activities of a midwife, *EU Second Midwifery Directive 80/155/EEC* cited in NMC (2004))

- People with special/additional needs – what they might need to know/want to know:

   (i) physical, sensory, learning disabilities (see McKay-Moffat 2007: 85–89 and 127–128)

   (ii) ethnic groups (especially if first language is not English)

   (iii) travellers

   (iv) socio-economically/educationally disadvantaged

   (v) teenagers

   (vi) substance abusers

- Aids to learning:

   (i) non-threatening environment

   (ii) mutual respect

   (iii) enthusiasm

   (iv) enjoyment

   (v) variety of methods

   (vi) topics selected by the group

- Attention span (possibly only 10–20 minutes) – therefore reinforce oral information with written

Student activity

- Note midwives' opportunities for offering individualised parent education
- Identify availability/format of sessions in your area (including private sector)
- Are special/additional needs being catered for?
- Consider your own educational needs in order to provide parent education
- Further reading: Deane-Gray (2004); Smith and Nolan (2009); Svensson and Barclay (2009)

Partogram completion

Commenced when labour established – speedy reference to progress in chart form with common information:
- Name, age, address, next of kin, religion, case sheet number
- Special instructions
- Routine observations recorded:
  - Temperature, pulse, blood pressure
  - Vaginal examinations – cervical dilatation, station of the head
  - Frequency/strength of uterine contractions
  - Liquor/loss *per vaginam*
  - Reaction to pain
  - Drugs administered/method of analgesia

May enable early recognition of deviations from normal and appropriate action.

Student activity

- Familiarise yourself/practise completing partogram used in your unit
- Further reading: Lavender *et al.* (2008); Vincent (2003)

Perineal repair

See **Perineal/surrounding area trauma**.

Part of a midwife's role (after instruction) to suture episiotomies/uncomplicated perineal tears – obstetrician's role if complicated.

Aim

- Aseptic technique
- Ideally repaired promptly – secures homeostasis/prevents oedema/ infection
- Delay ? makes procedure more difficult
- Minimise discomfort
- Align tissues correctly
- Reduce infection/deep vein thrombosis risk

Preparation

- Trolley with:
    (i) appropriate instruments
    (ii) antiseptic solution
    (iii) local anaesthetic (see **Episiotomy**, Anaesthetic) – unless effective epidural in place
    (iv) suture materials – current evidence indicates polyglycolic acid as Vicryl Rapide® causes less discomfort (see Kettle *et al.* 2002)
- Good light source
- Explain procedure
- Entonox available prn
- Lithotomy poles
- Stool for midwife to sit on whilst suturing
- Woman – bladder empty/in lithotomy position
- Maintain privacy

Action

- Midwife scrubs/wears sterile gloves
- Vulva/perineum swabbed
- Identify extent of trauma (see Sultan & Kettle 2007)
    (i) vagina examined – tear/episiotomy apex identified
    (ii) rectal examination with little finger to identify any rectal tearing (medical aid prn)
- Change gloves before proceeding
- Perineum re-infiltrated prn (see NMC 2007)
- ? Vaginal swab/tampon inserted (maintains clear site)
- Suture methods in use (1 or 2):
    ○ Method 1:
        (i) beginning at apex – continuous suture to vaginal mucosa, knot tied aligning fourchette
        (ii) two/three interrupted sutures into deep perineal layers (avoiding rectal mucosa)
        (iii) interrupted/continuous subcuticular suture to skin

- ○ Method 2:
  (i) Continuous suture is used through all layers of tissue – less suture material/knots
  (ii) (see Kettle *et al*. 2002, 2007)
- Remove swab/tampon
- Ensure haemostasis
- Gentle rectal examination to ensure mucosa not caught
- Swab vulva/perineum
- Dry pad applied
- Legs gently lowered

Following suturing

- Mother made comfortable
- Repair explained
- Contemporaneous records (NMC 2009)

Student activity

- Identify suture material used in your unit
- Observe procedure
- Simulated practice
- Further reading: Baston (2004a); Carroli and Migninil (2009); Dahlen and Homer (2008); Kettle *et al*. (2002, 2007); Langley *et al*. (2006); Metcalf *et al*. (2006); Steen and Marchant (2007); Sultan and Kettle (2007); Thakar and Sultan (2009)

Perineal/surrounding area trauma

See also **Perineal repair**.
- Pelvic floor/vulval area injury:
  Spontaneous/surgical incision
- First-degree tear (laceration):
  Shallow wound involving fourchette skin only
- Second-degree tear:
  Skin and perineal muscle damage, possibly with deep muscles/vaginal mucosa involved

- Third-degree tear:
  Damage extends to anal sphincter
- Fourth-degree:
  Damage through sphincter into rectal mucosa
- Vaginal wall:
  Commonly posterior wall – vaginal mucosa ? muscle, ? without skin damage
- Labial tears:
  Superficial skin tears, often very painful
- Clitoral tears:
  Uncommon – very painful
- Cervical tears:
  Profuse bleeding likely
- Episiotomy:
  A surgical incision of perineal skin, superficial/deep muscle and vaginal mucosa, following local anaesthetic infiltration; enlarges vaginal orifice (opening) (see Carroli & Migninil 2009)

Aetiology – tears

- Rapid, uncontrolled birth of baby's head (no gradual tissue stretching)
- May occur with cephalic presentation or after-coming head of breech
- Large baby/broad shoulders
- Malpresentation, e.g. occipito-posterior
- Hand involvement, i.e. baby's hand at face/shoulder widens shoulder diameter
- Alternative positions for birth, e.g. 'all fours' (labial, anterior wall, clitoral tears)
- Weak scar tissue (previous childbirth/cervical surgery)
- Instrumental delivery

Indications for episiotomy

- To speed up delivery in fetal/maternal distress when head on the perineum
- Minimise intracranial trauma in prematurity/breech

- Seriously delayed second stage (? rigid, poorly stretching perineum)
- Reduces maternal effort in serious medical condition, e.g. cardiac disease
- Prevention of trauma to previous surgery, e.g. pelvic floor/bladder repair
- Maternal request

Prevention of trauma – antenatal

- Well-balanced, nutritious diet
- Good hygiene
- Early detection/treatment of infection
- Pelvic floor exercises
- Complementary methods, e.g. oral arnica; massage with essential oils (see Beckmann & Garrett 2006; Rule 7, NMC 2004, 2007)

Prevention – labour

- Careful VEs – avoid overstretching/trauma, e.g. from Amnihook during ARM
- Non-directed pushing in second stage (i.e. not Valsalva manoeuvre)
- Appropriate use/timing of episiotomy
- Consider maternal position during second stage
- Controlled delivery of the fetal head ('guarding the perineum') (see McCandlish 1999; McCandlish *et al.* 1998 and **HOOP study**)
- Avoid prolonged second stage – 'prolonged' definition controversial
- Skilled instrumental delivery

Management – initial

- First-degree/labial tears:
  - Only sutured if bleeding/extensive
  - Sutures cause discomfort
- Second-degree/vaginal wall:
  - Sutured following local anaesthetic (part of midwife's role)
  - Medical aid if tear is very ragged/complicated
  - ? Non-suturing – no consensus that this is correct action – may be woman's choice

- Suture material – current evidence and research: Vicryl Rapide® less discomfort
- Third-/fourth-degree:
  - Medical aid – senior obstetrician and anaesthetist
  - Repair in theatre under GA/epidural/spinal as appropriate
  - Prophylactic antibiotics
- Clitoral tear:
  - Medical aid – ? sutured
- Cervical tear:
  - Urgent medical aid – senior obstetrician and anaesthetist
  - Suturing in theatre under GA/spinal or epidural if present
  - Management of haemorrhage
- Episiotomy:
  - As for second-degree
  - Discuss/obtain consent during pregnancy or early labour (prevent litigation/assault charge) – (see Dimond 2006)
  - Record-keeping of discussions/reason for episiotomy

Management – postnatal

- Good hygiene facilitates healing
- Treat any infection
- Analgesic prn – e.g. paracetamol/combination, e.g. co-proxamol; diclofenac
- Stinging by urine – during micturition, position change; warm water application, e.g. using a jug, shower spray or bidet; application of a barrier, e.g. Sudocrem or Vaseline (anecdotal evidence) – NB: moist healing is faster than dry healing
- Application of cold compresses (see Steen & Marchant 2007)
- No consensus of evidence about other ways of aiding healing/relieving pain
- Alternative therapies e.g. homeopathic, essential oils

Complications

- Infection/wound breakdown
- Perineal pain/discomfort

- Long-term morbidity
    (i) pain and dyspareunia (painful intercourse)
    (ii) psychological trauma
    (iii) relationship difficulties
    (iv) rectocele – hernia (bulging) of rectum into vagina (weak muscles)
    (v) cystocele – hernia of bladder into vagina
    (vi) fistula – opening between vagina and bladder (vesico-vaginal); or vagina and rectum (recto-vaginal) leading to incontinence

Student activity

- Revise wound healing
- Note local policies regarding episiotomy and analgesia
- Elicit midwives' skills in preventing perineal trauma
- Further reading: Layton (2004); Premkumar (2005); Thakar and Sultan (2009)

Phenylketonuria (PKU)

See also **Heel prick**.

An inborn error of metabolism of the amino acid phenylalanine – high blood levels are toxic to developing brain tissue; the metabolite phenylpyruvic acid is present in the urine.

Aetiology

- Genetically inherited, (see Figure 27) autosomal recessive: i.e. both parents carry an affected gene; incidence 1:10,000 births
- Deficiency of enzyme phenylalanine hydroxylase, which converts phenylalanine to tyrosine (both needed for growth)

Diagnosis

- Guthrie or Scriver test or chromatography on peripheral blood (see **Heel prick**) as part of routine neonatal screening (with parental consent)
- Fetal DNA testing if parents are known carriers

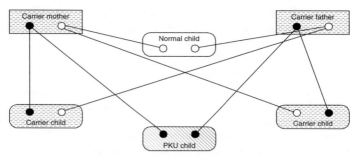

Each child has a 1:4 chance of having PKU at conception

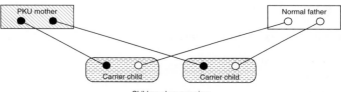

Children always carriers

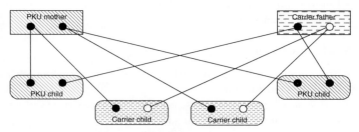

Each child has a 1:2 chance of having PKU at conception

Figure 27 Genetic inheritance, e.g. PKU.

Management

- Efficient screening system; result-monitoring part of local protocols
- Specialist paediatric unit referral/specialist dietitian
- Regular blood phenylalanine levels

• Low phenylalanine diet, i.e. special phenylalanine free infant formula + some breast milk/normal infant formula to provide the small amount of essential phenylalanine
• Liaison with health visitor/GP
• Phenylalanine-free supplements from weaning
• 'Special' low-protein foods available – bread, biscuits, flour, pasta
• Measured everyday foods, e.g. cereal, milk, potatoes; provide essential phenylalanine
• Diet now recommended to continue for life
• NB: women with PKU must resume very low phenylalanine diet 6 months before and throughout pregnancy, to avoid fetal brain damage
• Support from PKU society

Consequences – if untreated

• Growth retardation/restriction
• Microcephaly
• Brain damage
• Eczema
• Fair hair and skin extensively marked
• Urine has 'mousy' smell

Student activity

• Note your local policy regarding routine screening, including other tests on the same specimen
• Further reading: UK Newborn Screening Programme Centre Online: http://newbornbloodspot.screening.nhs.uk

PKU Society

A national support group for parents and children with PKU. Founded in 1973, it is the oldest PKU support society in the world.

NSPKU,
PO Box 26642, London N14 42F.
Tel: Helpline 0208 364 3010
Online: http://nspku.org

Phototherapy

See also **Jaundice**.
• Treatment for physiological/prematurity jaundice, ABO incompatibility
• No consensus in UK regarding bilirubin levels to initiate treatment (Rennie *et al.* 2009)
• Photoisomerisation reduces jaundice – blue-spectrum light converts fat-soluble bilirubin into less toxic water-soluble bilirubin for excretion
• Equipment commonly administers white and blue light:
    (i) Over the cot, portable light – baby's eyes covered
    (ii) Biliblanket – providing fibreoptic light – mat placed beneath/around baby – eyes uncovered/improved temperature maintenance

Aim

• Reduce serum bilirubin levels
• Maintain body temperature
• Prevent retinal damage
• Reassure/support mother

Preparation

• Phototherapy unit at mother's bedside
• Observation charts prn
• Adequate room/incubator temperature (baby nursed naked – check body temperature)
• Cover baby's eyes – secure eye pads, visor, shield over head

Action

• Baby naked under lights/on Biliblanket or Bilibed
• Ensure adequate eye protection
• Maintain observation chart
• Check that baby is comfortable
• Advise mother to remove baby for feeding, clean and undress, return
• No creams – danger of burning
• ? Extra fluids during treatment
• Bilirubin levels 8–12 hourly

- Continue phototherapy 36–48 hours
- Note skin rashes/diarrhoea
- When discontinued, continue bilirubin levels ? rise again
- Record discontinuation

Student activity

Further reading: Mills and Tudehope (2001); Pritchard *et al.* (2005); Rennie *et al.* (2009).

Placental examination

Performed quickly initially at delivery, then in more detail once mother/baby comfortable.

Aim

- Confirm placenta/membranes complete
- Identify abnormality
- Note number of placentae as potential indicator of zygosity in multiple births

Preparation

- Protected examining area
- Midwife wears gloves/plastic apron
- Good light source

Action

- Identify normality (Figures 28–30) or anomalies (Figures 31–36)
- Examine fetal surface:
  (i) Cord insertion – e.g. battledore (Figure 31) or velamentous (Figure 32) insertion
  (ii) Check for three vessels
  (iii) Note true/false knots
  (iv) Bipartite (Figure 33) or tripartite

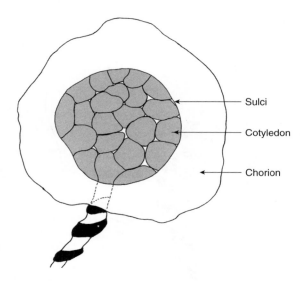

Figure 28 Normal placenta at term – maternal surface. Note cotyledons, sulci and chorion.

- Examine placental circumference:
  (i) ? Blood vessels into membranes/succenturiate lobes
  (ii) Peel membranes apart, viewing amnion/chorion (amnion peels back to cord, chorion to placental edge)
  (iii) Eliminate double chorion ring around circumference (circumvallate placenta)
- Examine maternal surface:
  (i) ? Normal colour/pale
  (ii) Consistency – ? normal, oedematous, calcification, 'grittiness', infarction
  (iii) Configuration – ? bipartite/tripartite
  (iv) ? Offensive smell
  (v) Push cotyledons together – identify torn/missing pieces
- Re-check chorion:
  (i) Extra (succenturiate) lobes (Figure 34) or holes
  (ii) Double fold (circumvallate placenta) (Figures 35 and 36)

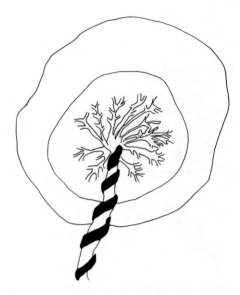

Figure 29 Normal placenta at term – fetal surface. Cord vessels supported by Wharton's jelly. Two arteries and one vein twist around each other. Vessels run deep into the placenta and extend over the surface.

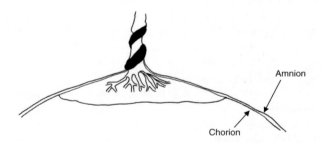

Figure 30 Normal placenta – lateral view showing two membranes. The chorion ends at the edge of the placenta. The amnion peels back to the cord.

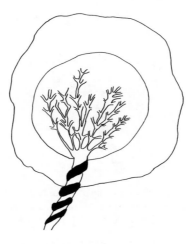

Figure 31 Abnormal insertion of the cord: Battledore insertion. Cord is inserted at the edge of the placenta. Danger of snapping during controlled cord traction (CCT).

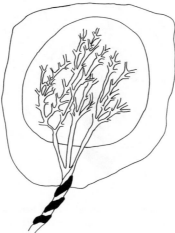

Figure 32 Abnormal insertion of the cord: velamentous insertion. Vessels travel through the membranes to be inserted into the placenta. Danger of haemorrhage if the vessels lie over the cervical os (vasa praevia) and the membranes rupture. Membranes may tear and cord separate during CCT.

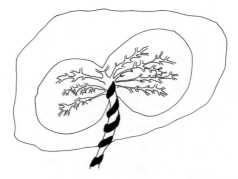

Figure 33 Abnormal placenta – bipartite placenta. Two lobes of varying sizes with cord implanted between them. Danger of the cord snapping during CCT. One lobe may separate properly whilst the other is retained.

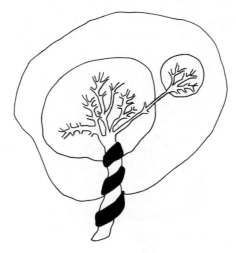

Figure 34 Abnormal placenta – succenturiate lobe. Blood vessels run through the membranes to an accessory lobe. Danger of haemorrhage from extra vessel if over cervical os (vasa praevia). Extra lobe may not separate and be retained in utero.

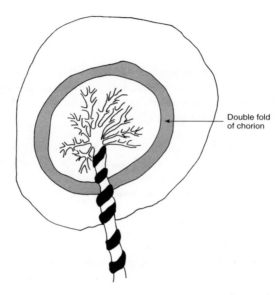

Figure 35 Abnormal placenta – circumvallate placenta. Double fold of chorion around the circumference of the placenta apparent on the fetal surface as a thickened white ring. Associated with placental abruption.

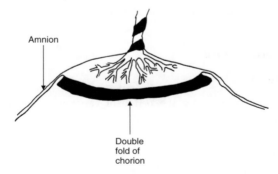

Figure 36 Lateral view of circumvallate placenta showing the amnion and the double fold of the chorion.

Multiple births

- Two/more separate placentae examined as previously
- If placentae fused together:
  (i) ? Examination to determine if one placenta, i.e. monozygotic (uniovular) or >1, i.e. non-identical twins – dizygotic (binovular)
  (ii) Two amnions/two chorions in twin pregnancy – ? = dizygosity (depends on when blastocyst divided)
- Method:
  (i) injecting fluid into cord and 'milking' it through placenta ? demonstrates whether the vessels go across – if yes, one placenta likely (monozygosity) – if no, two
  (ii) ? laboratory microscopic examination prn

Following examination

- Dispose safely according to policy
- If abnormality identified ? laboratory microscopic examination
- If stillbirth – placenta to laboratory for further examination
- Normal records

Student activity

- Seek every opportunity to examine placentae, especially if unusual
- Further reading: Ventolini *et al.* (2004)

Polyhydramnios

Definition

Excess amniotic fluid for the period of gestation – exact amounts difficult to specify.

Aetiology

- Idiopathic – i.e. not known
- Fetal abnormality, e.g. oesophageal atresia – fetus is not able to drink the liquor; anencephaly
- Macrosomic fetus

• Twin pregnancy – especially uniovular
• Rhesus isoimmunisation (Rh-negative mother with an Rh-positive fetus)
• Maternal diabetes – possibly resulting in fetal polyuria (excess urine) as a result of high blood sugar

Diagnosis

Abdominal examination

• Uterus feels large for dates
• Fetus may be difficult to palpate and FH difficult to auscultate
• A fluid 'thrill' can be felt across abdomen – lay a flat hand against the side of the woman's abdomen (with consent), tap the other side with tips of fingers and feel a 'ripple' effect on the inside of other hand

Ultrasound scan

Pockets of liquor are measured – amniotic fluid index; amounts vary in the literatuare but generally seem to be:
(i) individual pocket volume ≥8 cm deep
(ii) total depth of the four largest pockets >25 cm

Potential complications/risks

• Difficulty in abdominal palpation to define lie and presentation
• Separation of abdominal muscles (diastasis recti)
• Varicose veins – legs/vulva; risk of DVT
• May inhibit surfactant production in fetal lung (see **Respiratory distress syndrome**)
• Unstable lie
• Malpresentation, e.g. breech, face, shoulder
• Cord presentation or cord prolapse when membranes rupture
• Preterm labour/birth – due to uterine distension
• Placental abruption – if sudden decompression when membranes rupture
• Postpartum haemorrhage – due to inelastic myometrium (over-stretched)
• Amniotic fluid embolism

Management

• Explanation to mother – including action to take if membranes rupture
• Skin moisturiser/calamine to relieve stretching/itching
• USS for fetal anomaly
• Management of maternal diabetes if present
• Amniocentesis to drain some liquor – infection and preterm labour risk; liquor volume likely to re-occur
• Hospital admission to await labour if lie is unstable
• Controlled ARM (senior obstetrician) to induce labour/in early labour – examining fingers remain in vagina allowing slow draining of liquor to reduce risk of cord prolapse/malpresentation
• In labour be prepared for:
  (i) cord prolapse
  (ii) PPH – ergometrine may be needed for third stage
  (iii) amniotic fluid embolism (AFE)
• Paediatrician to examine baby promptly
• 10 FG nasogastric tube inserted prior to oral feeding to identify any oesophageal atresia (urgent surgical referral if suspected)

Student activity

• Revise formation of liquor
• Visit ultrasound department to see amniotic fluid index measuring – elicit definition of polyhydramnios in your maternity unit
• Further reading: Crafter (2009); Magann *et al.* (2000)

Postnatal care/examination – baby

See **Initial newborn examination**.

Aim

• Detect deviation from normal – structure, function, behaviour
• Reassure mother of baby's progress
• Support mother

- Health promotion/education e.g.
  - (i) Hygiene/general care
  - (ii) Breastfeeding/nutrition
  - (iii) Risk reduction for SIDS
  - (iv) Jaundice
  - (v) Vitamin K
  - (vi) Safe transport, e.g. by car
- Maintain accurate records (NMC 2009)

Preparation

- Neonatal chart
- Explain procedure/seek consent
- Mother present if possible and/or father
- Warm, private environment – maintain confidentiality
- Wash hands beforehand or use gel substitute if hands are clean – prevention of cross-infection

Action

- Head – ? swellings, bruising, fontanelle tension
- Eyes – ? discharge
- Mouth – ? *Candida* (thrush) – white plaques on tongue not removable
- Facial skin – ? marks/pustules
- Ears – ? discharge
- Take axillary temperature/undress baby
- Body skin – ? rashes, pustules, blisters
- Colour – ? jaundice, cyanosis, pallor
- Umbilical cord – ? redness, stickiness, pus around base – if separated is umbilicus clean, dry, bleeding?
- Buttocks/genitalia – ? rashes, redness, soreness
- Limbs – movement/position
- Note behaviour/muscle tone/reflexes
- Ask mother – about feeding, bowels, micturition, behaviour (fretful/distressed)

- Redress baby/give to mother
- Reassure mother by explaining findings
- Record accurately

Student activity

- Check local protocol for hand hygiene
- Revise neonatal thermoregulation
- Further reading: Demott *et al.* (2006); Trotter (2008)

Postnatal care – mother

- Should be culturally appropriate
- Able to meet additional needs, e.g. for women with disability; non-English speaking
- Encompasses maternal observations

Aim

- Offer support and guidance as required
- Advise woman of postnatal recovery
- Detect deviations from normal and seek medical aid (*Midwives' Rules and Standards*, NMC 2004)
- Early intervention preventing complications

Preparation

- Ensure privacy/comfort
- Prepare to meet additional needs, e.g. interpreter
- Postnatal records/charts available
- Equipment for vital sign measurement
- Explain examination/seek consent
- Woman lying almost flat for examination

Actions

- Vital signs:
    (i) TPR and BP prn – during first 6 hours postnatal
    (ii) TPR if temperature $\geq 38°C$/signs of infection – 4 hourly
    (iii) BP if diastolic $\geq 90\,mmHg$ 4 hourly

- Ask about:
    - (i) how she is feeling/any concerns/coping
    - (ii) bowels/micturition – ? burning/stinging
    - (iii) sleep/appetite
    - (iv) lochia/breasts/pain
- Check:
    - (i) general appearance, colour, demeanour
    - (ii) breasts prn, e.g. nipples ? cracks/bleeding; engorgement, mastitis
    - (iii) abdomen – palpate uterine fundus for consistency/position
    - (iv) lochia – observe colour, odour, consistency
    - (v) perineal sutures – mother lateral position ? healing/infection
    - (vi) legs – ? calf pain/tenderness, superficial phlebitis, oedema
- Discuss:
    - (i) normal changes physically/psychologically
    - (ii) self and infant care/feeding
    - (iii) early mobilisation
    - (iv) rest and recovery, e.g. postnatal exercises
    - (v) signs and symptoms of haemorrhage, infection, thromboembolism, depression
    - (vi) action to take if complications present
    - (vii) family planning/contraception
    - (viii) benefits of postnatal check about 6 weeks
- Accurately record in case notes
- Medical aid sought prn

The *Midwives' Rules and Standards* (NMC 2004) enables midwives to continue visiting mothers and babies after 28 days following delivery. This allows for:

(i) vital continuity of carer when actual/potential complications, e.g. postnatal depression

(ii) the midwife to conduct the 6-week postnatal examination (subject to adequate preparation)

Student activity

Further reading: Bick (2010); Demott *et al.* (2006); Moyzakitis (2004); Thompson (2004); Ward and Mitchell (2004); Yelland (2010).

Postnatal depression

A range of conditions, not always clearly defined or easily diagnosed, that include mild 'baby blues' (or third/fourth day blues); depression; puerperal psychosis; and post-traumatic stress.

Aetiology

- Not clear-cut – probably multifactorial
- May be present but undiagnosed during pregnancy
- Previous psychiatric history
- Existing neuroses, anxiety, phobia
- Socio-economic problems:
    (i) relationship difficulties
    (ii) poor support
    (iii) unplanned/unwanted pregnancy
    (iv) major life events, e.g. bereavement/moving house
    (v) financial/housing problems
- Obstetric history:
    (i) loss of previous pregnancy/baby
    (ii) complicated obstetric history
    (iii) difficult/traumatic pregnancy/birth (Laing 2001)
    (iv) a much-wanted pregnancy/baby – infertility treatment
- Hormonal imbalance – history of PMT increases risk

Baby blues

Signs and symptoms

Tiredness, weepy, feels emotionally low.

Management

- Effective support
- Rest/adequate sleep
- Information/reassurance

Depressive illness

Signs and symptoms

- Feelings of inadequacy/inability to cope
- Crying/feeling very 'low'
- Insomnia
- Lack of feelings towards baby
- Loss of libido
- Severe tiredness not relieved by sleep/rest

Diagnosis

- Often difficult – reluctant admission to feeling unwell
- Effective communication enables expression of feelings
- Listen to relatives (? behaviour change noticed)
- Edinburgh Postnatal Depression Scale (Webster *et al.* 2003) – 10 questions eliciting mother's feelings

Management

- Give mother time to talk – effective listening skills
- Debriefing of pregnancy and childbirth (present or past) experiences
- Medical aid – ? antidepressants
- Support from partner, relatives/significant person
- ? Postnatal support group
- Quality rest and sleep
- Exercise helps some women
- Alternative medicines (Mantle 2001)

Puerperal psychosis

Signs and symptoms

- Obviously very ill
- Altered perception of reality, e.g. of baby's abilities
- Delusions, e.g. baby dead; not given birth

- Confusion, e.g. about time/place
- Hallucinations (auditory/visual)
- Manic behaviour, e.g. obsessive cleaning
- Insomnia

Management

- Medical aid and hospital admission to psychiatric ward – preferably with baby
- Sedation reduces symptoms, e.g. chlorpromazine
- Appropriate treatment for diagnosis
- ? Electric convulsive treatment (ECT)
- Promote mother–baby attachment and parenting ability – initial close observation

Student activity

- Note your nearest psychiatric mother and baby unit
- Further reading: Bastos and McCourt (2010); Currid (2004); Davies (2003); Gibbon (2004); Henderson *et al.* (2003); Hendrick (2003); Kennedy and MacDonald (2002); Kightley (2008); Sumner (2002)

Postnatal exercises

- Exercise sheets commonly available
- Obstetric physiotherapist – ? visit wards for support
- Midwives' role to encourage frequent pelvic floor exercises

Aim

- Promote return of pelvic organs to pre-pregnancy state
- Prevent thromboembolic disorders
- Promote sense of well-being – may reduce postnatal depression
- Reduce risk of urinary/feacal incontinence
- Educate for future health

Preparation

- Postnatal exercises sheet for referral

- Mother empties bladder
- Ensure privacy

Action

(i) when recovered from delivery, encourage mobilisation

(ii) exercise gently initially – as strength returns, more vigorously; (NB: 3 months before progesterone effects subside)

(iii) feet – circular movements both directions; dorsiflex foot/wiggle toes

(iv) breathing – deep breathing/diaphragm used

(v) pelvic floor – tighten vagina and rectum, hold for 10 seconds/ release – repeat frequently when lying, sitting, standing

(vi) Buttocks – clench/relax, simultaneous tightening pelvic floor – repeat frequently

(vii) Hips – lying on bed, knees bent, feet to buttocks, swing knees side-to-side five times

(viii) Back/abdomen – all fours, arch back (big curve) – hold a few seconds/relax/repeat

(ix) Abdominal exercises – lying on back, knees bent, feet to buttocks – raise head/shoulders, touch right knee with left hand/ hold/relax/repeat with other hand

(x) When standing – try lengthening leg by raising hip, repeat on other side

Student activity

- Identify local policy/practise yourself
- Further reading: Bø *et al*. (2007); Hay-Smith *et al*. (2008); Whitford *et al*. (2007)

Post-partum haemorrhage – primary

Aetiology

- Failed contraction and retraction of the uterine muscle (the living ligature) to stop bleeding from the placental site
- Genital tract trauma from tear/cut, e.g. cervix, vagina, labia, clitoris, lower uterine segment, ruptured varicose vein

Predisposing factors

Previous history

- Grand(e) multiparity
- Obestity (Liston 2007)
- Over-distended uterus, e.g. multiple pregnancy, polyhydramnios, large baby
- Placenta accreta/percreta – increased incidence if previous C/S
- Retained products of conception – placenta, membranes or clots
- APH
- Anaemia
- Pre-eclampsia/eclampsia
- Inefficient uterine action/prolonged labour/oxytocic drugs in labour
- Abnormal uterus, e.g. in shape or with fibroid(s)
- Drugs, e.g. anaesthetics, tocolytics (uterine relaxants) in preterm labour
- Infection
- Inversion of uterus
- Mismanaged third stage, e.g. inappropriate manual stimulation of uterus

Birth

- Rapid uncontrolled birth
- Maternal expulsive effort (pushing) before cervix is fully dilated
- Difficult instrumental delivery or before cervix is fully dilated
- Episiotomy on a thick perineum

Prevention/minimise risks

- Treat anaemia, pre-eclampsia; prevent eclampsia, infection
- Identification of placenta accrete/percreta by USS or MRI (Liston 2007)
- Effective/appropriate labour care especially when risks identified, e.g.:
    (i) hospital birth
    (ii) blood to laboratory for save serum

(iii) IV cannula inserted, ? IVI

(iv) prevent prolonged labour, exhaustion, dehydration, full bladder

(v) appropriate use of oxytocics, including third stage

(vi) obstetric registrar at delivery

(vii) A/N guidance/preparation for woman who will refuse blood products

(viii) early warning scoring system (see **EWS/MOEWS** in Section 1; Clutton-Brock 2007)

Management

See Figure 37.

Complications of PPH

• Anaemia

• Shock/collapse – renal damage/failure, or Sheehan's syndrome (see subsequent entry)

• DIC

• Psychological morbidity, e.g. post-traumatic stress (see **Postnatal depression**)

• Hysterectomy – leading to inability to have more children

• Death – see Liston (2007)

Student activity

Further reading: Clutton-Brock (2007); Lewis (2007); Liston (2007).

Post-partum haemorrhage – secondary

Aetiology

• Retained products of conception, i.e. placenta or membranes

• Retained blood clots

• Infection

• Fibroid(s)

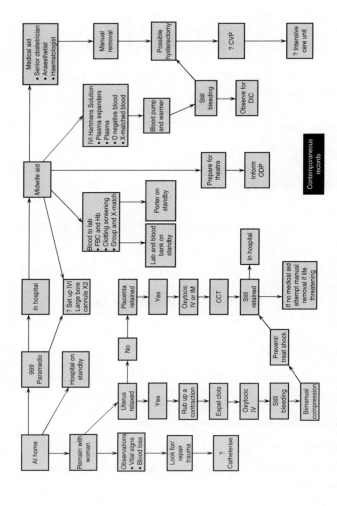

Figure 37 Post-partum haemorrhage – primary.

Signs and symptoms

- Subinvolution of uterus
- Tender uterus
- Lower abdominal pain/discomfort
- Heavy lochia ? clots, membrane, placental tissue
- Offensive lochia
- Low grade pyrexia +/− tachycardia
- General malaise (feeling unwell)

Management

See Figure 38.

Pregnancy-induced hypertension (PIH) and pre-eclampsia

Terms often used synonymously, but can be viewed as distinct.
- *PIH*

Hypertension due to pregnancy, i.e. a BP of 140/90 or an increase in diastolic 15–20 mmHg above usual (e.g. booking recording) on two occasions 24 hours apart (NB: if diastolic normally 60, a rise to 80 is significant)
- *Pre-eclampsia*
  - Potential eclampsia (fulminating pre-eclampsia = eclampsia imminent)
  - No clear consensus on definition
  - Commonly there is significant proteinuria (not due to UTI) and raised BP as above (NB: eclampsia may occur with normal BP) and ? significant oedema (e.g. facial)

Onset

- Commonly >32 weeks ? earlier; ? <20 weeks if hydatidiform mole (see Section 1)
- Condition variable in speed/progression

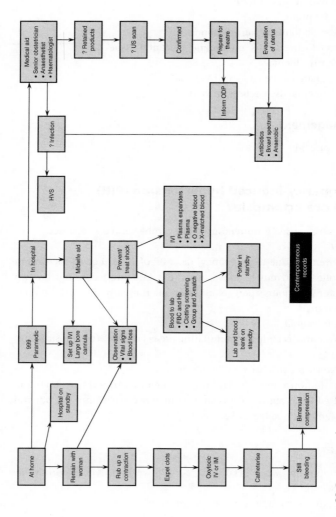

Figure 38 Post-partum haemorrhage – secondary.

Aetiology

- Not clear-cut; associated with a gravid uterus – resolves after delivery
- Possibly multifactorial/multi-system – including central nervous system and coagluation processes
- Possibly superimposed on existing high BP
- Hypotheses:
    ○ oxidative stress from high levels of circulating free radicals causing maternal vascular malfunction (see Rumbold *et al.* 2008)
    ○ placental influence
    (i) placental bed ischaemia, i.e. poor uterine artery flow, with high utero-placental resistance, due to poor implantation of trophoblast
    (ii) one or more factors from placenta transferred into maternal circulation, damaging blood vessels' endothelium; spasm raises BP; leaky vessels cause oedema
    ○ hormonal imbalance, e.g. prostaglandins (see Duley *et al.* 2007)
    ○ renin/angiotensin imbalance
    ○ immunological factors
    (i) commoner in primigravidas (sensitivity to 'foreign' genetic material)
    (ii) previous pregnancy (even aborted) offers some protection (sensitivity lowered)
    (iii) can occur (possibly for first time) if pregnant by new partner
    ○ maternal genetic factors – often familial, i.e. mother/sister had condition

Pre-disposing factors

Primigravida	Grand(e) multigravida	Multiple pregnancy
Very young	>35	Obesity
Social class V	Rhesus isoimmunisation	Hydatidform mole
Diabetic	Previous PIH/pre-eclampsia	Ethnicity

(See Duckitt & Harrington (2005); Hernández-Diáz *et al.* (2009)).

Management

Prevention

- ? Low-dose aspirin (inhibits platelet aggregation in placental site) (see **CLASP trial**, Duley *et al.* 2007)
- Dietary modification:

    (i) evening primrose oil or fish oil and/or calcium (balance prostaglandins) – inconclusive

    (ii) vitamin C 1000 mg + vitamin E 400 IU daily from early pregnancy (lowers circulating free radicals) – controversial; unproven (Rumbold *et al.* 2008)
- Magnesium sulphate (see Duley *et al.* 2003; **MAGPIE trial**; Neilson 2007)

Pregnancy

Regular monitoring of all women – they generally feel well until fulminating pre-eclampsia; therefore information to all women during pregnancy on recognition/action to take:

- Diastolic <100 *no* proteinuria or symptoms:

    rest at home, midwife checking BP and urine; ? self-monitoring
- Diastolic <100 + proteinuria/symptoms:

    admission
- Diastolic >100 +/− proteinuria or symptoms:

    admission
- Systolic 160 or more (must be considered significant – see Neilson 2007):

    admission

After admission

- Depends on severity of condition – intensive care may be needed (maternity unit/ICU)
- Note general condition including temperature/pulse
- BP 4 hourly or as frequently as every 15–20 minutes
- Fluid balance – particularly urine output ? catheterise (hourly measurement)

- IVI, ? CVP, nil orally
- Urinalysis for protein – ? 24-hour urine for total protein
- MSSU to exclude UTI
- Regular blood tests, e.g. 12–24 hours, for:
  - (i) FBC
  - (ii) coagulation studies
  - (iii) renal function – U & E; creatinine
  - (iv) liver function – liver function tests, enzymes, AST (see Section 1)
  - (v) magnesium levels if administered (antidote calcium gluconate)
- Control of BP, e.g.:
  - (i) methyldopa (Aldomet)
  - (ii) labetolol
  - (iii) hydralazine IM or IV for rapid control
- Prevention of convulsions, e.g.:
  - (i) magnesium sulphate (see Neilson 2007)
  - (ii) phenytoin
  - (iii) diazepam
- Assess fetal well-being
  - (i) movements
  - (ii) abdominal examination
  - (iii) CTG daily
  - (iv) USS and biophysical profile

Labour/delivery

- Induction of labour/caesarean section (NB: clotting screening available)
- Specific management if preterm
- Hospital (consultant unit) birth advisable – informed consent if woman wishes to remain at home (notify supervisor of midwives – NMC 2004)
- Senior obstetrician/anaesthetist
- Careful monitoring:
  - (i) hourly BP
  - (ii) continuous CTG

(iii) fluid balance (NB: Syntocinon antidiuretic properties avoid fluid overload)
- Adequate analgesia (epidural useful – lowers BP) to avoid stress from pain
- Be prepared for possible complications, e.g.:
    (i) ? haematologist/blood laboratory on standby
    (ii) drugs/equipment available
    (iii) paediatrician at delivery or on standby
    (iv) ? neonatal unit on standby
- Syntocinon for third stage (not Syntometrine – vasoconstriction effect of ergometrine increases BP – NB: recommendations of Neilson 2007, i.e. *no Syntometrine in cases where no BP recorded during labour*, e.g. rapid birth without labour care)

Postnatal

- Continue observation of BP (haemoconcentration may cause rise in BP)
- Eclampsia risk for 48 hours (in rare cases later)
- ? Continue antihypertensives

Complications

- *Fulminating pre-eclampsia* = imminent eclampsia
    ○ Recognition:
        – Headaches, retinopathy, visual disturbances
        – Renal damage
            (i) proteinuria
            (ii) oligouria
            (iii) raised blood urea
        – Hepatic damage
            (i) abdominal/epigastric pain (blood under liver capsule)
            (ii) vomiting (NB: ? misdiagnosing less serious conditions)
            (iii) jaundice – raised liver enzymes and AST (see Section 1)
- *Thrombocytopenia* – i.e. low platelets due to consumption – possible DIC
- *Haemolytic anaemia*

- *HELLP syndrome*
  - (i) **H**aemolysis
  - (ii) **E**levated **L**iver enzymes
  - (iii) **L**ow **P**latelets (Sibai 2004a)
- *Placental abruption/APH* – possible DIC
- *Myocardial infarction* (heart attack)
- *CVA* (cerebrovascular accident – stroke)
- *Adult RDS*
- *Eclampsia*
- *Death*
  - 18 noted in *Saving Mothers Lives 2003–2005* (Neilson 2007: 72)
- Mid-trimester miscarriage
- Placental insufficiency
  - Nutrient and O_2 deficiency leading to IUGR; fetal hypoxia; IUD
- Preterm delivery
- Perinatal death

Student activity

- Revise normal BP regulation mechanisms/changes antenatally
- Note non-pregnancy causes of hypertension
- Note your local management policies for PIH/pre-eclampsia
- Further reading: Draycott *et al.* (2000); Duley *et al.* (2003); Morley (2004)

Pre-labour or premature rupture of membranes (PROM)

See also **Preterm labour** and **Preterm baby**.

Incidence

Approximately 2–17% – many cases ? unrecognised.

Aetiology

- Unclear – known risk factors
- Previous history PROM

- Cervical surgery, e.g. cone biopsy
- Unhealthy placenta
- Antenatal procedures, e.g. amniocentesis
- Uterine trauma – accidental; violence
- Lower genital tract infections, e.g. *Trichomonas*, group B streptococci, *Staphylococcus aureus*, group B streptococci in previous child
- ECV
- Smoking
- Hypertensive disorders
- Diabetes
- Malpresentation
- Polyhydramnios
- ? Coitus (? due to prostaglandins in semen/released from cervix)
- ? VE
- ? Other genital tract infections, e.g. gonorrhoea, yeasts (thrush), *Chlamydia*

Management

History

- Onset of loss, amount, colour, smell, blood
- Differentiate with incontinence of urine/leucorrhoea
- Gestation, LMP/USS
- Risk factors present

Present symptoms

- General condition, including pyrexia
- Vaginal loss
- Contractions
- Dysuria
- Other symptoms

Social situation

- Help/support needed enabling rest
- Identification of domestic abuse – offer of specialist support

Examinations

- General condition and vital signs
- Abdominal palpation
- Auscultation FH
- CTG

? Speculum VE for:

    (i) cervical and low vaginal swabs

    (ii) confirmation whether liquor present, ? nitrazine stick (not 100% reliable)

    (iii) note cervical dilatation

    (NB: *no* digital VE until labour begins – infection risk)

- USS:

    (i) biophysical profile

    (ii) abnormalities

    (iii) gestation

    (iv) weight estimation

- *If* 37 weeks or more and no complications/risk factors:

    (i) ? await onset of labour (24–48 hours)

    (ii) ? go home/return daily for review

    (iii) ? immediate induction or wait 24–48 hours (Syntocinon or vaginal Prostin)

    (NB: woman's informed choice – risk of infection rises >24 hours)

- *If* mother/baby at risk whatever gestation – expedite delivery
- *If* preterm PROM (i.e. before 37 weeks):

    ○ senior obstetric/paediatric medical aid

    ○ *if* 32 weeks or less, or baby estimated <2500 g, and delivery expected – mother in unit with NNICU (possible *in utero* transfer, i.e. of pregnant woman to appropriate unit)

    ○ *if* fetus not compromised, and delivery not expected – treat conservatively:

        (i) maternal rest – hospital

        (ii) observe for infection:

            – general condition

            – vital signs

            – blood for white cell count and ESR daily

            – fetal tachycardia (reliable >28 weeks)

(iii) CTG daily

(iv) ? tocolytics (inhibit contractions) – useful for *in utero* transfer

(v) ? antibiotics (controversial), e.g. ampicillin/penicillin G, IM, or erythromycin

(vi) ? home if liquor lessens – continue monitoring/screening

○ *if* 24–34 weeks/delivery expected, IM corticosteroids – see **Preterm labour**

Complications

- *Cord prolapse leading to*:
  ○ Hypoxia/birth asphyxia
  ○ Perinatal death
  ○ Long-term morbidity, e.g. cerebral palsy
  ○ Social/psychological trauma
- *Intrauterine infection leading to*:
  ○ IUD
  ○ Maternal infection/puerperal sepsis
  ○ Maternal/neonatal mortality/morbidity
  ○ Social/psychological trauma

Student activity

- Note your local policy and procedures
- Further reading: Kenyon (1995); Kenyon *et al.* (2004); Lindsay (2004)

Preterm baby

See also **Small-for-gestational-age baby (SGA)** and **Preterm labour**.

A baby born <37 completed weeks gestation – may also be small for gestational age (SGA).

(i) low birth weight <2500 g

(ii) very low birth weight <1500 g

(iii) extremely low birth weight <1000 g

Characteristics

Head

- Appears large in proportion to baby
- Fontanelles/sutures wide
- Skull bones soft
- Eyelids ? fused
- Pinna of ear soft/will remain folded

Length

Proportional to weight.

Limbs

- Thin
- Nails soft, usually short

Muscle tone

- Poor
- Arms/legs abducted

Chest

- Small and narrow
- Little/no breast tissue

Skin

- Red/pink, transparent – veins visible
- Lacks subcutaneous fat
- Lanugo (hair) present, depending on gestation
- Vernix often marked, depending on gestation

Abdomen

- Large
- Umbilicus may appear low

Genitalia

- Small
- Testes may be undescended
- Labia majora not covering minora

Behaviour

- Cry weak/absent
- Little activity
- Poor/no sucking/swallowing

Aetiology

- Often unknown
- Spontaneous/induced for maternal condition
- Pre-eclampsia/hypertensive disease
- APH
- Maternal disease, e.g.:
  (i) renal
  (ii) diabetes
  (iii) severe infection, especially UTI, including asymptomatic bacteriuria
- Cervical incompetence
- Smoking, drug, alcohol abuse
- Multiple pregnancy
- Polyhydramnios
- Rhesus incompatibility
- Higher incidence in:
  (i) malposition/malpresentation
  (ii) teenage pregnancy
  (iii) multiparas
  (iv) poor maternal nutrition
  (v) low socio-economic groups
  (vi) psychological factors, e.g. stress and anxiety; violence and abuse
  (vii) abnormal uterus, e.g. bicornuate
  (viii) repeated TOP – ? damaged uterus/cervix
  (ix) abdominal surgery, e.g. appendectomy; removal of ovarian cyst

Management – initial

(See also **Pre-term labour.**)
• Delivery in consultant unit with NNICU (? *in utero* transfer – experienced escort)
• Paediatrician at delivery
• Necessary resuscitation measures (see **Birth asphyxia**)
• Maintain body temperature (see **Hypothermia – neonatal**)
• Initial parent–baby contact
• Transfer to NNICU
• Assessment of gestational age (see **Dubowitz Score** in Section 1)
• Weigh and place in incubator
• Baseline observations via monitoring equipment:
  (i) temperature
  (ii) respiratory rate and oxygen saturations
  (iii) heart rate
  (iv) blood glucose (see **Heel prick**)
• ? IVI and/or arterial line (usually umbilical artery via cord stump)
• ? Intubation and ventilation
• ? Infection screening
• ? Prophylactic antibiotics
• Information and support to parents

Management – subsequent

(NB: may involve moral/ethical dilemmas for parents/staff – support essential.)
• Maintain respiration/oxygen levels
• Monitor vital signs
• Thermoregulation (see **Hypothermia – neonatal**)
• Monitor/maintain blood glucose
• Fluid balance
• Hygiene and prevention of infection
• Feeding:
  (i) parenteral (IVI)
  (ii) enteral (into gut via oral/naso-jejunal tube)
  (iii) intragastric (oral/nasogastric tube)
  (iv) oral

- Parental information/psychological support
- Parental participation in care is encouraged
- Consider individual cultural, religious, personal beliefs/values and needs
- Paediatric follow-up after discharge

Complications

- Perinatal/neonatal death
- Associated with specific congenital abnormalities
- Birth asphyxia
- Cerebral haemorrhage
- Persistent fetal circulation
- RDS/SDS (respiratory distress syndrome/surfactant deficiency syndrome)
- Hypothermia
- Hypoglycaemia
- Hypocalcaemia
- Jaundice
- Infection
- Anaemia
- Haemorrhagic disease
- Iatrogenic conditions (i.e. those due to treatment):
  (i) retinopathy
  (ii) bronchopulmonary dysplasia (BPD) – chronic respiratory disease (mechanical ventilation)
  (iii) necrotizing enterocolitis (NEC) – bowel inflammation, ischaemia and obstruction
- Long-term morbidity:
  (i) cerebral palsy
  (ii) motor/neurological impairment
  (iii) learning difficulties
- SIDS – increased risk

Student activity

- Revise fetal circulation/adaptation to extra-uterine life
- Compare/contrast characteristics of pre-term/SGA baby
- Further reading: Saigal and Doyle (2008); Victoria *et al.* (2008)

Preterm labour

See also **Pre-labour or premature rupture of membranes (PROM)** and **Preterm baby**.

Labour commencing <37 completed weeks gestation.

Aetiology

- Spontaneous – see **Preterm baby**
- ? Low maternal progesterone (Lachelin *et al*. 2009)
- Induced because of:
  (i) fetal compromise
  (ii) IUD
  (iii) maternal condition (see **Induction of labour – alternative and natural; and Induction of labour – medical**)

Prevention

- Optimise maternal well-being – pre-conception and antenatal:
  (i) nutritious diet
  (ii) socio-economic factors
  (iii) infection screening and treatment for asymptomatic bacteruria (NICE 2008a)
  (iv) management of maternal conditions
  (v) family spacing
  (vi) stop smoking/substance use
- ? Cervical suture for incompetent cervix

Management

- Admit to consultant unit with NNICU (? *in utero* transfer – experienced escort)
- Obstetric medical aid (senior)
- History:
  (i) booking and antenatal
  (ii) gestation
  (iii) present general condition – including signs of infection
  (iv) vital signs
  (v) contractions
  (vi) vaginal loss

- Examinations:
  - (i) abdominal
  - (ii) FH auscultation, CTG (30 minutes)
  - (iii) ? digital VE by obstetrician if membranes intact
  - (iv) speculum VE by obstetrician if membranes ruptured (see **Pre-labour or premature rupture of membranes [PROM]**)
  - (v) urinalysis – routine dip stick and MSSU
  - (vi) blood – FBC, ? group/save serum
  - (vii) ? USS
- Treat underlying cause
- ? Prophylactic antibiotics (see **ORACLE trial**)
- IVI – sodium lactate (Hartmann's solution) – rapid hydration ? decreases contractions
- *If* 24–34 weeks and no contraindications:
  - IM corticosteroids to mature fetal lungs:
    - (i) dexamethasone 6 mg IM × 4 doses 12 hours apart; or
    - (ii) betamethasone 12 mg IM × 2 doses 24 hours apart (NB: blood glucose levels will significantly rise in diabetics)
  - deliver in unit with NNICU (? *in utero* transfer – experienced escort)
- *If* no contraindications, e.g. compromised fetus, severe vaginal bleeding and 24–34 weeks, delay delivery long enough for corticosteroids to be effective – ? tocolytics (controversial)

Tocolytic	*Administration route*	*Possible side-effects*
(a) Ritodrine (Yutopar)	IVI	Tachycardia and palpitations vomiting, headache tremors, anxiety
(b) Salbutamol (Ventolin)	IVI	Tachycardia and palpitations vomiting, headache tremors, anxiety
(c) Terbutaline	SC/IVI	Tachycardia and palpitations vomiting, headache tremors, anxiety

(d) Magnesium sulphate (calcium gluconate antidote)	IV bolus/IV	Respiratory arrest in high doses neuromuscular effects; monitor serum calcium and magnesium levels
(e) Indomethacin (inhibits prostaglandins)	oral/rectal	Gastrointestinal irritant; headaches and dizziness ?closure of fetal ductus arteriosus
(f) Nifedipine (effective prolonged use)	oral	Facial flushing, headaches, oedema, constipation, hypotension

Complications

- Preterm baby
- Instrumental/operative delivery (short- and long-term maternal consequences)
- Social and psychological implications

Student activity

- Revise the initiation of labour
- Note your local policy and protocols
- Further reading: Goldenberg *et al.* (2008); Lachelin *et al.* (2009); RCOG (2002, 2004)

Primary Care Trusts (PCTs)

The PCTs replaced primary care groups. They are responsible for improving public health at local level by planning and commissioning health services. This includes ensuring that adequate staff and services are available from hospital and community services. This incudes GPs, dentists, mental health-care, Walk-In Centres, NHS Direct, patient transport (including emergency), population screening, pharmacy and opticians. The integration of health and social care systems is included in their role.

Student activity

Consider the role of the midwife in public health. Further reading: Edwards *et al.* (2005).

Prolonged labour – first stage

There is no consensus of opinion about time, but commonly 12–24 hours in established labour is considered prolonged (NB: avoid including time during the latent phase of the first stage).

Aetiology

- Inefficient/incoordinate uterine action
- Malposition/malpresentation
- CPD
- Non-engagement of presenting part
- Cervical dystocia, e.g. due to scarring from surgery or TOP
- Psychological factors leading to hormonal/chemical imbalance, e.g. oxytocin and catecholamines
- Entering birthing pool too early, e.g. before cervix is 4–5 cm dilated

Management

- Identify possible cause
- Mobility and upright position
- Psychological support
- Adequate analgesia
- General physical care
- Observations:
  - fluid balance
  - vital signs
  - urinalysis
  - progress:
    - (i) contractions
    - (ii) descent of presenting part – abdominally/on VE

(iii) cervical dilatation

(iv) ? continuous electronic monitoring

- Augmentation/acceleration of labour as appropriate
- Caesarean section as appropriate, e.g. for CPD

Complications

- Maternal stress:
  - (i) anxiety
  - (ii) frustration
  - (iii) anger
  - (iv) tiredness or exhaustion
  - (v) emotional
- Greater pain sensitivity
- Maternal distress:
  - (i) physical and emotional exhaustion
  - (ii) raised temperature and BP
  - (iii) dehydration and oligouria
  - (iv) ketosis
  - (v) vomiting
- Intrauterine infection
- Ruptured uterus
- Risk operative/instrumental delivery
- Risk PPH
- Fetal hypoxia
- Early neonatal infection
- Perinatal mortality
- Neonatal/infant morbidity
- Post-traumatic stress/long-term psychological trauma

Prolonged labour – second stage

- Without progress in the active stage:
  - >30 minutes for multipara
  - >1 hour for primigravida
- The timing is traditional, but debatable; a longer time is increasingly acceptable if fetal and maternal conditions are satisfactory and progress is being made

Aetiology

- Inefficient uterine action
- Poor maternal effort due to:
  - (i) exhaustion
  - (ii) epidural
  - (iii) fear/pain
- Full rectum/bladder
- Rigid perineum
- Contracted pelvic outlet/CPD
- Persistent OP position
- Deep transverse arrest
- Malpresentation

Management

- Support and encouragement
- Change in maternal position, e.g.
  - (i) left lateral
  - (ii) upright
  - (iii) 'all-fours'
- Close observation of FH (minimum every 5 minutes – ? continuous)
- Medical aid:
  - (i) obstetrician
  - (ii) paediatrician
  - (iii) anaesthetist
- Syntocinon infusion
- ? Episiotomy
- ? Instrumental delivery – forceps or ventouse
- ? Caesarean section

Student activity

Note your local policies on definitions and management of prolonged labour.

Pruritus

Itching – abdominal, vulval, general.

Aetiology

Abdominal

- Unclear
- General skin stretching
- Striae gravidarum, i.e. pregnancy stretch marks
- Hormone links, e.g. corticosteroids

Vulva

- Infection, e.g. yeasts, i.e. *Candida* (thrush); bacteria
- Sweat rash
- Glycosuria

General

- Allergic reaction – food; antibiotics; blood transfusion
- Infection, e.g. viral rash
- Cholestasis (see earlier entry) – commonly hands and feet

Management

Abdomen

- Little effective prevention
- Moisturising cream popular
- Oil-based calamine lotion if severe

Vulva

- Identify organism – HVS, vulval swab and appropriate treatment
- Effective hygiene
- Urinalysis/investigate glycosuria
- Cotton underwear
- Avoid tights/tight-fitting clothes

General

- Identify cause
- Withdraw allergen

- Antihistamine for allergic reactions
- Investigate possible cholestasis
- Local preparations to relieve itching, e.g. calamine lotion

Pudendal nerve block

(Not a midwife's role).
- Pudendal nerves supply external genitalia, perineum, lower vagina
- Obstetrician's role ? prior to instrumental delivery/perineal repair
- Not always effective
- Transvaginal approach is common – ischial spines are palpated/injection either side
- Perineal approach if presenting part very low

Aim

- Assist the doctor
- Support woman/partner
- Maintain accurate records (NMC 2009)

Preparation

- Delivery trolley with pudendal block pack (includes guarded needle, e.g. Oxford needle)
- Local anaesthetic, e.g. lignocaine (lidocaine) 0.5%/1.0%
- Syringes
- Empty woman's bladder
- Entonox available

Action

- Explain procedure
- Assist opening packs/drawing up local anaesthetic
- Place legs in lithotomy position
- Offer Entonox/support
- Safely dispose of needles on completion
- Ensure that records are completed

Pulse taking

Aim

• Palpate/count peripheral pulse (commonly radial; ? temporal; ? carotid in neck) i.e. the contractions of left ventricle of heart
• Accurately record

Preparation

• Explain procedure
• Client seated/resting
• Watch/clock with second hand
• Observation chart/records

Action

• Lift arm/place two fingers over wrist's inner border
• Locate pulse/count for 1 minute
• Note rate, if irregular, weak, bounding – record
• Inform client of findings
• Medical aid if abnormal
• Record (NMC 2009)

Relaxation techniques

• Encouraged/practised during pregnancy since 1930s – Grantley Dick-Reid proposed that stress/tension increased labour pain, causing more stress/tension; but relaxation exercises break cycle – also information reduced fear/tension
• Psychoprophylaxis – a series of relaxation/breathing exercises
• Relaxation exercises helping us cope with everyday living can be beneficial in pregnancy/labour

Aim

• Encourage total body relaxation during pregnancy
• Increase body awareness
• Provide sense of well-being/confidence

Preparation

- Small group teaching ideal
- Mats/pillows
- Advised loose clothing
- Maintain privacy
- Woman lying comfortably supported by pillows

Action

- Working from head to toes, encourage awareness of posture/tension present, e.g.:
  - head – jaw tension
  - frowning – conscious effort to smooth brow, relax jaw
  - tongue comfortable in mouth/teeth not grinding
  - neck – relaxed, head supported by pillows
  - shoulders – note tension, relax/let pillows support
  - arms – note muscle tension, let arms fall loosely by sides
  - hands – let fingers relax, palms open, wrists loose/floppy legs/feet the same
  - abdominal muscles – relaxed buttocks/pelvic floor
  - total body relaxation
- Encourage concentration on breathing; note different levels, i.e.
  - deep breathing using diaphragm
  - shallow breathing using intercostal muscles
  - panting using upper respiratory muscles
- Practise deep breathing/total relaxation – maintain awareness of feeling of full relaxation
- Gradually increase body tension/return to sitting position/upright position

Student activity

Attend local session/practice exercises.

Respiratory distress syndrome (RDS) (Surfacant deficiency syndrome [SDS])

- Respiratory condition – alveoli inflation difficult/impossible
- Commoner in neonates than adults

Neonatal

Aetiology

- Lack of surfactant (surface activating or active agent) causes alveoli to collapse on expiration, requiring great respiratory effort for the next breath
- NB: phospholipids lecithin and sphingomyelin are precursors to surfactant – present in liquor (see **LS ratio** in Section 1)

Predisposing factors

Prematurity, especially <34 weeks:
- Caesarean section
- APH
- Diabetic mother
- Hypoxia/acidosis
- Maternal drug abuse

Prevention

- Delay preterm delivery until lungs mature
- Promote lung maturity/surfactant production – maternal IM dexamethasone or betamethasone (corticosteroids) (see **Preterm labour**)
- Avoid perinatal hypoxia/acidosis
- Tight control on maternal diabetes antenatally
- Control maternal drug addiction

Signs

- Difficulty initiating normal respiration
- Breathing difficulties in first few hours after birth
- Grunting sound on expiration
- Hypotonia (poor muscle tone)
- Sternum/intercostal muscles drawn in; flaring of nostrils
- Cyanosis
- Tachycardia
- Reduced breathing sounds
- X-ray picture

Management

- Paediatrician
- Admission to NNICU
- Intubation/mechanical ventilation
- Monitor/maintain blood gases; temperature; blood glucose levels
- Replacement surfactant therapy (Stevens *et al.* 2005)
- Parental information/support

Complications

- Cerebral haemorrhage
- Pneumothorax (air in chest cavity)
- Persistent fetal circulation
- Sepsis
- DIC
- Death
- Long-term morbidity, e.g. bronchopulmonary dysplasia (BPD) (long-term O_2 need)
- Neurological disorders

Adult

Aetiology

- Profound hypoxia – due to hypotension; haemorrhage; DIC
- Mendelson's syndrome

- Hypertensive disorders
- Sepsis

Management

- Medical aid – senior obstetrician/anaesthetist
- Treat underlying cause
- Assisted ventilation
- Intensive care unit

Complications

- Maternal death – six during 2003–2005 linked to other conditions (Lewis 2007)
- Long-term morbidity – physical, social, psychological

Student activity

Further reading: Lewis (2007); Stevens *et al.* (2005).

Resuscitation of newborn

See **Birth asphyxia**.

Retained placenta

See **Delivery technique**, third stage of labour.
- The placenta is considered retained:
  - (i) after 30 minutes in active third stage
  - (ii) after 1 hour in physiological third stage
- It may be:
  - (i) wholly or partially separated – danger of PPH
  - (ii) trapped in the cervix or uterus – danger of PPH
  - (iii) still adherent to the uterus – PPH less likely

Aetiology

- Uterine inertia:
  - (i) failure of contraction and retraction of myometrium to separate and expel placenta

(ii) may follow incoordinate uterine action, prolonged or precipitate labour
- Full bladder:
  Inhibits uterine function and/or delays descent of placenta
- Mismanagement of third stage:
  (i) use of CCT before Syntometrine is effective
  (ii) 'fiddling' with the uterus – causes inertia or incoordinate uterine action
  (iii) delay in using CCT following Syntometrine – causes placental entrapment by closed cervix
- Uterine abnormality: e.g. bicornuate uterus increases risk
- Constriction ring – spasm of uterine muscles above lower segment inhibits expulsion
- Pre-term labour – particularly if induced
- Adherent placenta:
  (i) partially, e.g. by infarcts
  (ii) partially/wholly due to being:
    - attached *to* myometrium (placenta accreta)
    - attached *into* myometrium (placenta increta)
    - attached *through* myometrium (placenta percreta)

Management

See Figures 39 and 40.

Manual removal

- An obstetric procedure, may be undertaken by a midwife in an emergency (see Activities of a midwife, *EU Second Midwifery Directive 80/155/EEC* cited in NMC (2004))
- Morbidly adherent placenta may be retained for natural absorption

Complications

- Post-partum haemorrhage
- DIC
- Perforated uterus

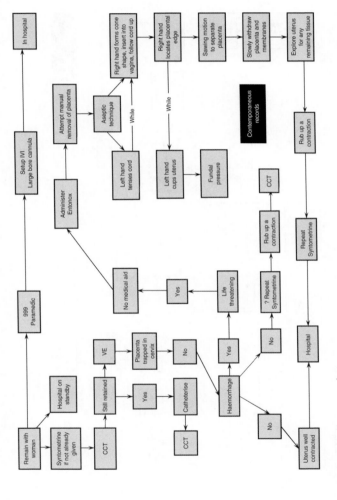

Figure 39 Retained placenta – at home.

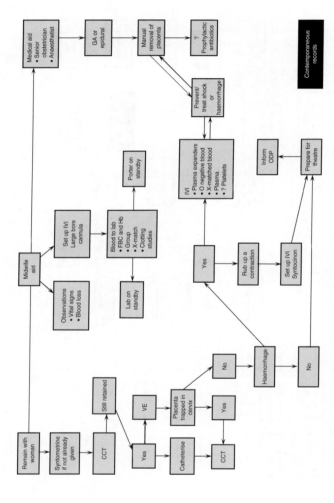

Figure 40 Retained placenta – in hospital.

- Sepsis
- Death
- Hysterectomy (especially if morbidly adherent)/subsequent infertility

Student activity

- Note your local policy/procedures for management in community/hospital settings
- Engage in simulated emergency drills

Retinopathy of the newborn

(Retrolental fibroplasia)

Characteristics

- Abnormal development of blood vessels in the eye – may:
  (i) regress
  (ii) lead to local or complete retinal detachment – long-term visual impairment or blindness
- Five stages – from demarcation of vascular and avascular zones to complete retinal detachment
- Additional blood vessel abnormalities
- Clouding of the vitreous humour – plus disease – increase the severity of condition

Aetiology

- Not fully understood – ? multifactorial
- Pre-term/very low birth weight babies susceptible
- Noted in stillborn/full-term infants
- Oxygen therapy implicated, i.e. when levels are too high, particularly in premature infants
- Hypothetical causes:
  (i) toxic oxygen – O_2 therapy combined with blood transfusion/iron; neonatal hypoxia/anoxia, e.g. in bradycardia/apnoea
  (ii) intrauterine hypoxia, e.g. in pre-eclampsia

(iii) intraventricular haemorrhage at delivery or after birth
(iv) inability to synthesise prostaglandins – linked to toxic oxygen
(v) light, e.g. 24-hour brightness while in incubator

Prevention

- Minimise risk of hypoxia/trauma
- Avoid prematurity
- Strict neonatal blood gas monitoring/control of O_2 levels
- Reduce/discontinue O_2 as soon as possible – avoid rapid change
- Minimal handling/procedures avoid O_2 concentration change
- Rapid response to bradycardia/apnoea

Management

- Early screening by ophthalmologist
- Laser therapy or cryotherapy to minimise the destructive consequences of the condition
- Paediatric follow-up

Complications

- Visual impairment, e.g. tunnel vision, due to:
  (i) damaged retina
  (ii) retrolental (behind lens) fibrous mass
  (iii) cataracts; glaucoma
- Myopia (short sight)
- Nystagmus (rapid eye movements)
- Strabismus (squint)
- Photophobia (sensitivity to light)
- Microphthalmia (small eyes)
- Blindness

Student activity

- Elicit your maternity unit screening policy
- Further reading: Clarkson (2001, 2002); Siderov (2008)

Safe Motherhood Initiative

With the aim of reducing worldwide maternal mortality and morbidity, the World Health Organisation (WHO) launched the Safe Motherhood Initiative in 1987. Key target areas are improvement in education/social standing for women; improvement in health services, including family planning; better education for midwives (especially untrained traditional birth attendants [TBA]), including how to manage emergency situations, e.g. PPH, eclampsia and obstructed labour. Individual countries employ specific solutions to meet their unique needs.

Sexually transmitted infection (STI)

See also **Antenatal screening** and **Infection – maternal** and **Infection – neonatal**.

Infections spread by sexual contact:

(i) Viral, e.g. hepatitis A, B, C; human papilloma virus (genital warts); *Herpes simplex* type 2; HIV

(ii) Bacterial, e.g. gonorrhoea; *Gardnerella*

(iii) Protozoal, e.g. *Trichomonas vaginalis*

(iv) Spirochaete, e.g. syphilis

(v) Parasitic, e.g. *Chlamydia trachomatis*

(vi) Fungal (yeasts), e.g. *Candida* (thrush)

Sheehan's syndrome

Hypopituitarism, i.e. poor/failed pituitary function.

Aetiology

A rare anterior pituitary necrosis following prolonged shock (APH/PPH).

Signs and symptoms

- History
- Failed lactation

- Secondary amenorrhoea, i.e. no menstruation following childbirth
- Diminished thyroid/adrenal function (lethargy, feeling cold, coarse skin/hair)
- Libido loss
- Diminished secondary sexual characteristics

Management

Hormone replacements – thyroxin, corticosteroids, HRT.

Complications

Infertility – associated with hormone reduction/failure.

Shoulder dystocia

- A complex clinical phenomenon
- An obstetric emergency – no classic definition
- Failure of spontaneous vaginal delivery of fetal shoulders after head has been born (without use of specific manoeuvres) – commonly, anterior shoulder is obstructed behind the symphysis pubis/posterior shoulder below sacral promontory

Risk factors

Large fetus – especially >4000 g – may be influenced by:
(i) maternal age >35
(ii) large maternal birth weight (not usually enquired about at booking)
(iii) maternal obesity
(iv) diabetes (gestational or existing) often causes macrosomic baby i.e. >4000 g

Pelvic abnormalities

(i) narrow outlet
(ii) platypelloid shape
(iii) small pelvis

Maternal immobility/position in labour

(i) recumbent position – narrows outlet by inhibiting 'give' of pelvic joints and extension of coccyx

(ii) epidural analgesia – immobility and lack of pelvic floor tone leads to poor shoulder descent/rotation

Incidence

Often quoted as 1–2%; depends on categorisation, i.e. are shoulders delayed or impacted?

Management

See Figure 41.

Skill, judgement and the individual case dictate method/manoeuvre used, for example:

- **McRoberts manoeuvre**

With the mother in the dorsal position her knees are placed in an exaggerated knees–chest position; normal delivery of shoulders may now be possible

- **All-fours position**

This can facilitate the delivery of the posterior shoulder first, which releases the trapped shoulder, enabling delivery

- **Wood's or Rubin manoeuvres** (usually by obstetrician)
  - These involve internal rotation of the fetal shoulders through 180 degrees
  - Suprapubic pressure can be applied to release the trapped shoulder

- **Zavanelli manoeuvre** (by obstetrician)

Cephalic replacement followed by caesarean section

Complications

Baby

- Perinatal mortality/morbidity
- Birth asphyxia/hypoxia

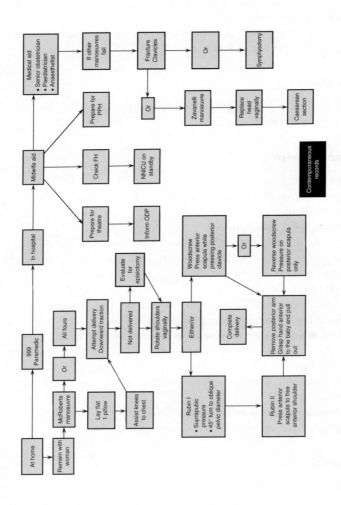

Figure 41 Shoulder dystocia.

- Erb's palsy
- Brachial plexus injury
- Fractured clavicle or humerus – especially when traction is used

Mother

- Uterine rupture – especially if fundal pressure is used
- Intrapartum or post-partum haemorrhage
- Trauma – perineal; pelvic floor; cervical; haematoma formation
- Long-term morbidity:
  - (i) physical
  - (ii) psychological
  - (iii) social
  - (iv) sexual

Student activity

- Note your local procedures
- Engage in simulated manoeuvres
- Further reading: Guerewitsch *et al.* (2005); Mahran *et al.* (2008); O'Leary (2008); RCOG (2005, 2007); Squire (2002)

Sickle cell disease

See **Haemoglobinopathies**.

Small-for-gestational-age baby (SGA)

See also **Preterm baby** and **Intrauterine growth restriction (IUGR)**.

A baby below the 10th percentile for gestation, i.e. with IUGR (NB: baby may also be preterm); may be symmetrical or asymmetrical.

Characteristics

	Asymmetrical	*Symmetrical*
(1) Head	Normal for gestation	Small for gestation
	Large for weight	Normal for weight
	Fontanelles normal	Normal
	Skull bones hard	Skull bones hard
	Eyes open	Eyes open
(2) Length	Long for weight	Normal for weight
(3) Limbs	Thin for size	Normal for size
(4) Muscle tone	Normal	Normal
(5) Chest	Ribs clearly visible	Normal
	Breast tissue normal	Normal
(6) Skin	Loose, dry, scaling, cracked	Normal
	Nails long and firm	Nails long and firm
	Normal colour or meconium-stained	Normal colour
	Lack subcutaneous fat	Lack subcutaneous fat
(7) Abdomen	Hollow	Normal
	Cord dries and separates early	Thin cord separates early
(8) Genitalia	Normal	Normal
(9) Behaviour	Alert and lively	Alert
	Very hungry	Normal appetite
	Eager to suck	Normal sucking

Aetiology

Asymmetrical growth restriction

Occurs from third trimester – linked to diminished placental function due to:

(i) pre-eclampsia and hypertensive disorders

(ii) smoking

(iii) multiple pregnancy

(iv) infarction after separation, e.g. APH, threatened abortion

Symmetrical growth retardation/restriction

- Develops early in pregnancy, e.g. due to:
  - No identifiable cause (often)
  - Intrauterine infection
  - Maternal conditions:
    (i) systemic/genital tract infections
    (ii) blood disorders, e.g. anaemia, haemoglobinopathies
    (iii) chronic respiratory disease
    (iv) severe renal or cardiac disease
    (v) metabolic disorders, e.g. PKU
    (vi) medications, e.g. steroids, cytotoxics, phenytoin (see **Epilepsy**)
    (vii) substance abuse, e.g. alcohol, drugs
    (viii) malnutrition
    (ix) low socio-economic status
- Fetal conditions:
  (i) inherited factors, e.g. small build, chromosomal abnormalities
  (ii) congenital abnormalities, e.g. cardiac, renal
  (iii) intrauterine infections, e.g. rubella and other viruses, toxoplasmosis

Management – initial

- Delivery in consultant unit with NNICU (? *in utero* transfer – experienced escort)
- Paediatrician at delivery
- Necessary resuscitation measures (see **Birth asphyxia**)
- Thermoregulation (see **Hypothermia – neonatal**)
- NNICU or transitional care prn
- Weighed
- Base-line observations:
  (i) temperature
  (ii) respiratory rate – ? oxygen saturation

    (iii) heart rate

    (iv) blood glucose

- Information and support to parents

Management – subsequent

- Depends on condition
- Early feeding
- ? Blood glucose monitoring
- ? Infection screening
- Thermoregulation
- Monitor elimination
- Hygiene and prevention of infection
- Continue information and support for parents
- Paediatric follow-up after discharge

Complications

- Symmetrically growth-retarded – poorer prognosis
- Perinatal/neonatal mortality
- Neurological damage from hypoxia (before, during, after birth)
- Persistent fetal circulation
- Increased risk of SIDS
- Long-term physical/neurological morbidity, e.g. motor function/behaviour

Student activity

- Compare/contrast SGA/preterm baby
- Further reading: Victoria *et al.* (2008)

Smoking and pregnancy

Reasons women may smoke:
- Aids coping with – anger, stress, frustration, poor home conditions
- Peer pressure/fashion
- Gives confidence
- Physical/psychological dependence

- Something to do/habit
- Keep weight down
- Give break/time for self
- ? Only purchase made for herself
  Tobacco smoke:
  Contains thousands of chemicals (metabolites found in urine, saliva, cervical secretions) – most dangerous being:
- *Carbon monoxide (CO)*
  - Hb has a 200 times greater affinity for CO than O_2 (results in O_2 deficiency)
  - CO elimination from fetus slower than from mother
  - Increases blood viscosity (thick, sticky); leads to:
    (i) increased thromboembolic disorders
    (ii) poorer circulation – poor O_2 perfusion – IUGR
    (iii) poor uterine circulation – IUGR
- *Nicotine*
  - Reaches brain 10 seconds after inhalation
  - Increases adrenaline/decreases noradrenaline – mood alteration:
    (i) lowers aggression/stress
    (ii) increases tolerance
    (iii) causes feeling of excitement
    (iv) improves vigilance, concentration, speed/reaction time
    (v) heightens arousal
    (vi) lowers efficiency of food metabolism
    (vii) lowers appetite
  - Aids release of catecholamines from adrenal and nerve cells, resulting in:
    (i) increased heart rate/vasoconstriction
    (ii) increased O_2 consumption
    (iii) increased use of free fatty acids – hypoglycaemia
    (iv) lower placental blood flow/fetal breathing movements
- *Polycyclic aromatic hydrocarbons*
  Interfere with normal enzyme transport.
- *Hydrogen cyanide*
  (i) broken down into thiocyanate
  (ii) lowers blood pressure (less risk of PIH)

(iii) lowers B_{12} levels
(iv) ? combines with amino acids – less protein available for fetal growth

Complications

Short term

- Usually dose-related, i.e. number smoked daily/amount inhaled
- ? Link with passive smoking
- Lowered fertility
- Low oocyte production in assisted conception
- ?? Sperm damage
- Spontaneous abortion rate considerably higher, more likely in fourth to seventh month
- Most harm to fetus after fourth month
- Lower PIH but more perinatal deaths if it does occur
- Placenta praevia/abruption commoner
- Low birth weight – approximately 170–200 g; lower if mother drinks alcohol
- Increased perinatal mortality – cessation improves statistics
- ? Increased congenital abnormalities
- Increased risk of PROM
- Increased preterm delivery
- Increased fetal distress in labour; therefore operative/instrumental delivery
- Lactation capacity down
- Tobacco metabolites in breast milk
- Early baby weaning commoner in smoking mothers

Long term

Increased risk of:
- SIDS
- Infant mortality
- Respiratory disease, e.g. bronchitis, pneumonia, asthma
- Glue ear/hearing difficulty
- Hospitalisation

- Retarded physical/mental development
- Vascular-related disease in later life
- Leukaemia – twice the risk
- Increase in all cancers
- Twice as likely to smoke in later life

Management

- All smokers expect to be asked about smoking
- Be sensitive and non-judgemental – a dogmatic approach ? causes reluctance to attend
- Elicit knowledge about smoking and pregnancy
- Ask why she smokes
- Ask how she feels about smoking – would like to stop/not

Not willing to stop

- Correct misinformation
- Explain how smoking is harmful to the baby
- Offer other information only if she wishes
- Warn about likelihood to be asked again
- Complete accurate records of discussion

Considering stopping/wishes to stop

- Correct misinformation
- Explain how smoking is harmful to the baby
- Explore potential difficulties in stopping
- Elicit available family/friends support
- Ask her what would help her to give up
- Offer possible ideas to help, e.g.:
    - (i) consider what it would be like not to smoke
    - (ii) choose a day to stop
    - (iii) dispose of remaining cigarettes, matches, lighter, ashtray
    - (iv) make one room/whole house no smoking zone
    - (v) ask for help from family/friends; they may join in!
    - (vi) change routine to avoid usual smoking situations

    (vii) keep hands busy
    (viii) save the money towards baby clothes/equipment
- Offer continued support yourself
- Offer information about local/national support groups
- Inform her that her progress will be questioned during next visit
- Complete accurate records of discussion

Student activity

- Review your local policy on smoking in pregnancy information-giving.
- Find leaflets available in your unit
- Identify any local smoking cessation support groups
- Further reading: Bauld *et al.* (2009); Ebert *et al.* (2009); Lorente *et al.* (2000); McCowan *et al.* (2009); Osadchy *et al.* (2009); Wisborg *et al.* (2001)

Stillbirth

See **Intrauterine death**.

Stillbirth and Neonatal Death Society (SANDS)

A national charitable organisation since 1981 based in London, with local branches and members, offering help and support to bereaved mothers and families following miscarriage, stillbirth or neonatal death. The society has highlighted the needs of bereaved parents and issued guidelines for service providers and practitioners on ways of improving services.

    SANDS,
    23 Portland Place,
    London,
    W1B 1LY.
    Tel: Monday–Friday 020 7436 5881 – helpline 9.30 a.m. – 5.30 p.m.
    Monday–Friday 020 7436 7940 – head office 10 a.m. – 5 p.m.
    Fax: 020 7436 3715
    E-mail: support@uk-sands.org
    Web site: http://www.uk-sands.org

Strategic Health Authorities (SHAs)

The SHAs have the responsibility for strategic development and quality assurance in local NHS health services. They link Department of Health directives and national priorities with local service provison, e.g. improving cancer services and standards for the prevention of methicillin-resistant *Staphylococcus aureus* (MRSA) infection. Since 2006 the number of SHAs in the United Kingdom has been reduced from 28 to 10.

Substance-abusing mother and baby

Substances

(Many abusers are poly (many) drug users):
- Alcohol
- Amphetamines, e.g. speed; ecstasy (E)
- Cocaine; crack cocaine
- Narcotics, e.g. heroin, morphine
- Cannabis
- Smoking (see **Smoking and pregnancy**)
- Tranquillisers/sedatives, e.g. valium, temazepam
- Volatile liquids/gases

Methods of consumption

- Ingestion, e.g. tablets, alcohol
- Inhalation, e.g. tobacco smoke, smoked heroin, vapours from glue/butane gas
- Transdermal, e.g. skin patches
- Rectally, e.g. ecstasy
- Snorting, e.g. cocaine
- IV, e.g. heroin; some non-IV substances, e.g. temazepam, methadone

Aetiology

Commonly multifactorial:
- Socio-economic/psychosocial factors
- Peer pressure

- Cultural influences
- Poor parenting
- Lack of education

Complications – general

- Poor nutrition
- Behavioural malfunction
- Criminal activity:
  (i) prostitution (to pay for habit)
  (ii) sexual promiscuity
  (iii) violence
- Infections:
  (i) general (poor resistance)
  (ii) STIs
  (iii) IV transmitted, e.g. hepatitis, HIV, septicaemia (shared equipment, non-aseptic technique)
- Injury/death:
  (i) accident
  (ii) overdose
  (iii) hyperpyrexia (ecstasy)
  (iv) inhaled vomit
- Circulatory:
  (i) thrombophlebitis
  (ii) abscess or fibrosis at IV site
  (iii) thromboembolism
  (iv) cardiac arrhythmias/arrest
- Respiratory:
  (i) nasal damage (cocaine)
  (ii) asthma/bronchitis
  (iii) respiratory arrest

Complications – maternal

- Amenorrhoea/infertility
- Unrecognised/unacknowledged pregnancy
- Late/non-booking/poor attender antenatally

- Absent family/friends support
- Unable/unwilling to attend parent education
- Poor knowledge about pregnancy, childbirth, parenting
- Poor nutritional status, lack of vitamins, iron and folic acid
- Preterm labour

Complications – baby

- Spontaneous abortion
- Chronic fetal hypoxia – IUGR
- Fetal distress in labour/perinatal hypoxia
- Preterm birth/low birth weight
- Perinatal death
- Congenital abnormalities due to:
  (i) early intrauterine infection
  (ii) fetal alcohol syndrome
- Neonatal thermoregulation difficulties
- Neonatal drug addiction/withdrawal syndrome
- Prolonged physical/mental morbidity

Management

- Pre-conception (ideally) to detoxify/improve nutritional status
- Antenatal:
  (i) early booking – non-judgemental approach
  (ii) thorough history – including substance(s) used (not always accurately given)
  (iii) antenatal screening (especially infection, e.g. hepatitis, HIV, STI prn)
  (iv) nutritional advice
  (v) monitoring fetal well-being (diminished fetal breathing movements on USS)
  (vi) referral/liaison – drug management team/midwife; ? methadone (liquid narcotic substitute) or buprenorphine (Subutex) (sublingual tablet) opiod replacement programme – slowly decreasing doses to lessen withdrawal symptoms/illicit drug use (sudden withdrawal ? fetal distress, abortion, preterm labour)

(vii) encourage regular antenatal attendance, including parent education

(viii) liaison – social services/health visitor; ? attendance at case conference(s)

- Labour:

  (i) continuous CTG

  (ii) pethidine ? ineffective – epidural suitable analgesia

  (iii) paediatrician at delivery

  (iv) no neonatal naloxone (Narcain) ? cause sudden withdrawal symptoms

  (v) ? neonatal unit on standby

- Postnatal:

  (i) breast-feeding ? suitable depending on individual circumstances – methadone levels low in breast milk (Jansson *et al.* 2007) (NB: breast milk alcohol levels = maternal plasma alcohol levels)

  (ii) continue liaison – multiprofessional team prn

  (iii) additional support aids parenting skill development

  (iv) continue methadone schedule

- Neonate:

  (i) remains with mother if possible

  (ii) special care unit prn

  (iii) possible withdrawal symptoms:

  – tremors, jitters, convulsions

  – diarrhoea

  – sneezing

  – high-pitched cry/very unsettled

  – sweating

  – feeding difficulties

  (iv) treat/manage withdrawal symptoms:

  – sedatives, anticonvulsants, ? morphine

  – prevent dehydration

  – comfort/soothing

  (v) ? infection screening

  (vi) information/support mother

  (vii) ? long-term paediatric follow-up

Student activity

• Find out your local policy on management of mother/baby
• Further reading: Dryden *et al.* (2009); Jansson *et al.* (2007); Meyer *et al.* (2007); Wright and Walker (2007)

Sudden infant death syndrome (SIDS)

(Cot death).

The sudden death of an infant unexplained by history or post-mortem examination.

Incidence

• 305 deaths in the United Kingdom in 2007 – rate 0.39 per 1000 live births (FSID 2009)
• 76% fall in the rate in babies ≥ normal birth weight since 'Reduce the Risk' campaign in England and Wales in 1991 (FSID 2009)

Aetiology

• Unclear – ? multifactorial, ? combined factors during a vulnerable time
• Possibilities – genetic vulnerability; brainstem abnormalities of serotonin
• Occurs any time from birth – incidence peaks at 2–3 months, but low incidence beyond 9 months

Risk factors

• Low birth weight (LBW)
• Preterm birth
• Multiple birth
• Male – 1.3 times higher incidence (FSID 2009)
• Maternal age < 20 at time of birth – especially without supportive partner/living alone (FSID 2009)

- High maternal parity – especially if <25 years
- Short interval between pregnancies – <6 months
- Low parental socio-economic status
- Low parental educational achievement
- Parental unemployment
- Smoking – maternal smoking during pregnancy (Wisborg *et al.* 2001) (increases with number of cigarettes and with paternal smoking)
- Infant passive smoking
- Sleeping prone (on the front)
- Overheating – excess bedding/clothing; room temperature; fever (NB: temperature control mechanism inefficient); illness

Prevention/risk reduction

- Improved socio-economic factors – including family spacing, maternal health
- Ideally, prevent preterm and LBW babies
- Stop smoking before/during pregnancy; avoid baby's passive smoking
- Avoid overheating:
    (i) sleep supine (on back) in own cot in parents' room
    (ii) room temperature 16–20°C
    (iii) head uncovered; baby's feet at cot bottom prevent slipping under bedding
    (iv) avoid direct heating – hot water bottle/radiant heat
    (v) no excess clothing/soft bedding, especially if unwell/fever
- Breast feeding (DH 2007b; Vennemann *et al.* 2009)
- Use of dummy (pacifier) once breastfeeding established (DH 2007b)
- Monitor baby's general health/prompt medical attention prn
- Parents taught CPR

Student activity

- Note your local policies/available literature for parents
- Further reading: DH (2007b); Moon *et al.* (2007); Vennemann *et al.* (2009)

- For latest information see Foundation for the Study of Infant Deaths Online: http://www.fsid.org

Symphysis pubis pain/sacro-iliac pain

- Pain at/surrounding symphysis pubis joint, +/− sacroiliac joint pain: increasingly diagnosed but still under-reported
- A potentially debilitating condition impacting on quality of life

Aetiology

- Pregnancy hormone link: i.e. progesterone and relaxin soften joint cartilage and relax supporting ligaments (pelvis 'gives' more room for birth)
- Occurs during pregnancy, labour, puerperium
- Joint inflammation, swelling; symphysis pubis diastasis or dysfunction (SPD) leads to joint movement
- Squatting position during pregnancy, labour, delivery strains joint
- Unaccustomed exercise, especially involving leg abduction (opening out)
- Large baby
- CPD
- Abnormal presentation
- Precipitate labour
- Difficult delivery
- Careless leg abduction into lithotomy position (NB: epidural may mask joint strain)

Signs and symptoms

- Joint/groin pain, ? radiates to thighs/lower back
- Sensation of joint movement
- Difficulty walking/weight-bearing, climbing stairs, getting into bed/bath
- Waddling gait (walk)
- Separation may be seen on X-ray/USS

Prevention

- Avoiding unaccustomed exercise/leg abduction (NB: care in aqua-natal exercises)
- Avoid heavy lifting/use correct lifting technique
- Abdominal support for woman with lax muscles
- Correct management of labour, especially placing into lithotomy position

Management

- Depends on symptom severity
- Bed rest – ? hospital, in most comfortable position – ? supported left lateral (NB: DVT prevention)
- Obstetric physiotherapist referral
- Muscle strengthening exercises
- Pelvic support/binder – Tubigrip/Tubipad
- Regular analgesia – low-dose opiods may be necessary
- Adduct legs (knees together) for movement between standing position and bed/chair
- Minimise weight-bearing – wheelchair, elbow crutches, walking frame
- Shower (use chair), not bath
- Mobilisation as condition allows
- Help/support at home
- Consider labour/delivery position – have a 'dry run' – ? left lateral /'all-fours'
- Careful movement/lithotomy position during epidural, avoiding strain/worsening

Complications

- ? Caesarean section if severe
- Long-term social/psychological morbidity (chronic pain)

Talipes equinovarus

A congenitally abnormal position of one/both feet.

Aetiology

- Muscle and tendon contraction
- ? Genetic origin
- Commonly from intrauterine position – breech, oligohydramnios (low liquor volume)

Recognition

Part of midwife's initial neonatal examination.

Management

- Depends on severity
- Paediatric/physiotherapist referral
- Passive exercises (teach mother)
- Splinting or plaster cast
- Surgery

Complications

- Delayed recognition prolongs treatment
- Difficulty/inability walking

Student activity

Further reading: Hart *et al*. (2005).

TAMBA – Twins and Multiple Birth Association

A national charity set up in 1978 providing information to professionals and information and support to parents with twins or multiple pregnancy/births.

TAMBA,
2 The Willows,
Gardner Road,
Guildford, Surey,
GU1 4PG.

Tel: 01483 304442 Monday–Friday 10.00 a.m. – 4.00 p.m.
Fax: 01483 302483
Email: enquiries@tamba.org.uk
http://www.tamba.org.uk/html/home.htm

Teenage pregnancy

- Pregnancy in under-18s
- Early teenage pregnancy = baby born to girl of 16 years/younger
- Potentially has a major effect on physical, social, emotional well-being (see DH 2004); controversy about direct link to adverse obstetric outcomes – links may be indirect i.e. due to lifestyle rather than age
- UK teenage pregnancy rates continue to rise – highest in Europe (WHO 2007)
- Government initiatives developed to lower rate (see *Every Child Matters*, Dcsf 2003)
- Lack of sex education/knowledge may not be the reason for unplanned pregnancy – midwives are in a position to offer teenagers support, advice, referral to appropriate agencies
- Specific parent education sessions may be provided for teenagers

Common issues

- Delay in recognising pregnancy – late booking
- Concealed pregnancy – no one to talk to
- Termination of pregnancy – 50.6% of pregnancies in under-18s and 61.9% in under-16s in England in 2007 (Dcsf 2007)
- Late TOP – increased physical/psychological risks
- Higher risk of pregnancy complications:
  - (i) anaemia
  - (ii) PIH/pre-eclampsia/eclampsia – especially if obese
  - (iii) APH
  - (iv) preterm birth/LBW babies/IUGR
  - (v) CPD
  - (vi) fetal abnormalities/stillbirth

- Socio-economic/psychological problems:
  (i) high-risk activities – smoking, alcohol, drugs
  (ii) poor nutrition
  (iii) poverty – especially <16 (unable to claim benefit themselves)
  (iv) rejection – family/partner
  (v) incomplete education – affects long-term employment – poverty trap
  (vi) family stress/marital break-up/disputes over child care/rearing/ domestic violence or abuse

Student activity

- Identify local initiatives to support/educate pregnant teenagers
- Further reading: Bailey *et al.* (2004); Chen *et al.* (2007); Dcsf (2003; 2007); Dimond (2006); Kidger (2004); Paranjothy *et al.* (2009); Shakespeare (2004)

Temperature-taking

Aim

Identification of pyrexia (>37°C); hyperpyrexia (>40°C) or hypothermia (<35°C).

Sites

- Oral – accurate
- Rectal – accurate – higher reading than oral
- Axilla – less accurate – lower reading than oral
- Skin – ? accurate – much lower reading than oral
- Ear (tympanic membrane) – accuracy possibly debatable (see Farnell *et al.* 2005)

Types of thermometer

- Mercury-in-glass – no longer considered safe
- Electronic digital – oral, skin, ear

- Chemical/disposable – oral, axilla, skin – probably not suitable for professional use
- Low reading

Preparation

- Explain procedure
- Ensure privacy prn
- Appropriate thermometer for site + disposable covers prn
- Gloves/lubricant for rectal
- Temperature chart

Action

Oral

- Unsuitable for neonate
- Eating, drinking, smoking avoided 20–30 minutes beforehand
- Apply disposable cover prn
- Gently insert bulb into posterior sublingual (under tongue) pocket
- Retained until ready (electronic); for minimum 1 minute (chemical)
- Remove, remove disposable cover, read
- Clean/disinfect according to local policy
- Chart results

Axilla

- Suitable for neonate
- Place thermometer in axilla centre
- Arm lowered and placed across chest
- Retained until ready (electronic); 3 minutes (disposable)

Rectal

- Unsuitable for neonate or those with rectal conditions
- Client turned on to side/knees bent
- With gloved hand, lubricate disposable cover on thermometer, gently insert into anus 3–4 cm
- Retain until ready

- Remove, remove disposable cover, clean thermometer and anal area
- Return client to comfortable position
- Continue as above

Skin (electronic)

- Suitable for neonate
- Select appropriate site (abdomen common)
- Fix with hypoallergenic tape
- Connect to recording apparatus/incubator temperature control
- Chart results

Tympanic

- Unsuitable for neonate
- Apply disposable cover to thermometer speculum
- Insert probe gently into outer ear canal
- Reading within 1–2 seconds
- Chart result

Student activity

- Note your local policies
- Further reading: Farnell *et al.* (2005); Harris (2009); Mains *et al.* (2008)

Tentorial tear

A torn tentorium cerebelli (a layer of the dura mater membrane between cerebrum and cerebellum).

Aetiology

- Sudden/excessive moulding of fetal skull during birth, because of:
    (i) OP position
    (ii) precipitate labour
    (iii) rapid second stage
    (iv) uncontrolled head of breech

- Large/extended head
- Prolonged labour
- Operative delivery
- Delicate skull – prematurity

Signs

- Birth asphyxia with slow/no recovery
- Hypotonia (floppy), ? followed by hypertonia (stiff)
- Signs of cerebral irritation:
    (i) irritability
    (ii) poor feeding
    (iii) lethargy
    (iv) vomiting
    (v) jittering/convulsions
    (vi) apnoea attack (stops breathing)
    (vii) shrill cry
    (viii) tense/bulging fontanelles

Management

- Paediatrician
- NNICU
- Gentle handling
- Monitor vital signs
- Stabilisation of blood gases and glucose, temperature
- Control convulsions
- IV fluids
- Konakion (vitamin K_1) 0.5 mg or 1.0 mg IV/IM
- Paediatric follow-up

Consequences

- Concurrent tearing of large vein (vein of Galen)
- Cerebral haemorrhage
- Neurological damage
- Long-term morbidity
- Neonatal death

Term breech trial

• A multicentre, international randomised controlled trial of planned caesarean section vs. planned vaginal delivery of the breech fetus at term, to identify the best approach to management. Began in January 1997, ending in July 2000. Centres included Argentina, Canada, Chile, Finland, India, the United Kingdom and the United States, with Canada funding and coordinating the project

• Inclusion criteria included pregnancy minimum of 37 weeks; frank (extended) or flexed (not footling) breech presentation; live fetus; no evidence of CPD

• Exclusion criteria included estimated fetal size of 4000 g or more and contraindications to vaginal delivery

• Results indicated that caesarean section to deliver the breech at term resulted in lower perinatal mortality and morbidity and no increase in serious maternal consequences

• Considerable debate continues about the research methodology and subsequent validity and reliability of results. See further reading

Student activity

Further reading: Bewley and Shannon (2007); Glazerman (2006); Hannah *et al.* (2000).

Thalassaemia

See **Haemoglobinopathies**.

Thrombosis and Thromboembolism

See **Deep vein thrombosis** and **Embolism**.

Thrombophlebitis

See also **Deep vein thrombosis**.

Inflammation of vein with clot formation – usually superficial vein and associated with **varicose veins**.

Signs and symptoms

- Painful red swelling over superficial vein
- May be oedema

Management

- Apply a supportive bandage
- Soothing agent such as glycerine and ichthyol applied
- Woman should rest with legs elevated
- No need to restrict movements and anticoagulant therapy not required

Transverse/oblique lie

Non-longitudinal lie of the fetus with shoulder presentation.

Aetiology

- Lax uterine/abdominal muscles (grand[e] multiparity)
- Placenta praevia
- Polyhydramnios
- Multiple pregnancy
- Abnormal uterus
- Uterine fibroid
- Abnormal pelvis

Diagnosis

- Abdominal palpation:
  - (i) fundus is low/abdomen broad
  - (ii) head is felt laterally
- Ultrasound scan

Management

- >32–34 weeks obstetric referral
- USS – identify cause/exclude abnormalities
- >37 weeks ? ECV
- Inform woman of urgent admission if SRM

- At term ? ECV and immediate induction of labour with Syntocinon
- ? ARM (senior obstetrician) once head enters pelvis
- Continuous electronic monitoring in labour
- Emergency caesarean section prn

Complications

- Obstructed labour
- Cord prolapse

Twins

See **Multiple pregnancy**.

Urinary tract infection – UTI

See also **Cystitis**.

Bacterial infection of the urinary tract (bladder, cystitis; kidney, nephritis or pyelonephritis), commonly by *E.coli* (normal bowel flora).

Aetiology in pregnancy

- Relaxation of smooth muscle of the ureters due to progesterone causes urinary stasis
- Short female urethra increases risk of ascending organisms from external genetalia, especially if personal hygiene is poor.

Aetiology in neonate

Susceptibility to transmission of organisms, especially if low birth weight.

Signs and symptoms

Adult	*Neonate*
General malaise (feeling unwell)	Jaundice
Vomiting	Vomiting
Pyrexia	Normal/unstable temperature

Abdominal/loin pain or tenderness   Diarrhoea
Frequency of micturition – ? painful
? Offensive urine
Haematuria (blood in urine)
Uterine contractions possible

Management

- History
- General observations – condition, temperature, pulse
- MSSU
- High fluid intake – oral/IVI
- Appropriate antibiotics (see **ORACLE trial** related to the prevention of **Preterm labour**)
- Uterine relaxants if danger of preterm labour
- Treat neonatal jaundice

Uterine inversion

A uterus partially/completely inside out – fundus above the cervix/protruding at vulva.

Aetiology

- Spontaneous – precipitate labour/poor uterine tone
- Third-stage mismanagement – excess fundal pressure/cord traction as uterus relaxed
- Short cord – pulls fundus down during the birth
- Manual removal of placenta – continued fundal pressure as the hand is removed from the uterus

Signs and symptoms

- Fundus visualised at vagina/felt on VE
- Severe pain
- Excessive bleeding/PPH

- No uterus palpated abdominally
- Shock – neurological (nerve/ligament traction) and/or haemorrhagic

Management – initial

See Figure 42.
- Replace the uterus manually – hydrostatic pressure may help
- Do not attempt to remove placenta

Management – subsequent

- Debriefing
- Encourage postnatal exercises

Complications

- Profound shock – renal damage; Sheehan's syndrome
- Sepsis
- Psychological trauma
- Anxiety in subsequent pregnancies

Student activity

- Note local policies
- Further reading: Kroll and Lyne (2002)

Uterine rupture

Complete

Perforation of the myometrium and perimetrium, with the fetus expelled through the uterine wall; placenta separates.

Incomplete

The perimetrium remains intact containing the fetus, and may stop the placenta from separating.

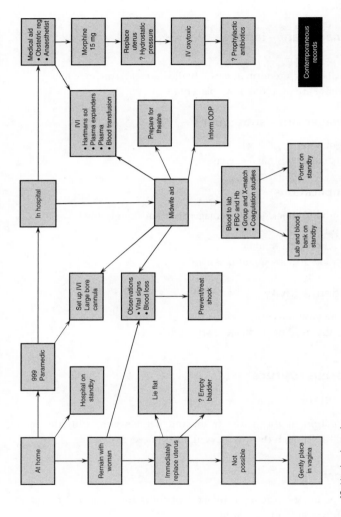

Figure 42 Uterine inversion.

Aetiololgy

(i) Cause unclear. One or a combination of:

(ii) Prostaglandin/oxytocic misuse

(iii) Weak scar tissue – previous surgery, e.g. caesarean section/uterine evacuation

(iv) Instrumental delivery – especially using Kielland's forceps

(v) Extended cervical tear

(vi) Severe placental abruption

(vii) Intrauterine manipulation, e.g. in shoulder presentation

(viii) Placental accreta (i.e. morbidly adhered to uterus)

Signs and symptoms

- Often dramatic with complete – possibly 'silent' with incomplete
- Severe constant abdominal pain
- Reduced contractions
- Vaginal bleeding
- Tachycardia
- Hypotension, shock and collapse
- Fetal distress
- IUD
- Fetal parts felt outside uterus
- Seen at caesarean section

Risk reduction

Woman with scar

- Senior obstetrician-led care (antenatal/intrpartum) recommended
- Hospital birth in a consultant unit recommended
- Avoid/cautious use of prostaglandins/oxytocic
- Close intrapartum fetal/maternal monitoring
- Early referral to senior obstetrician if symptomatic

General

- Appropriately used/managed prostaglandins/oxytocics (close fetal/ maternal monitoring – avoid complacency)

- Senior obstetrician for Kielland's forceps/intauterine manipulation – ? caesarean section safer
- Forceps delivery only when cervix fully dilated
- Avoid maternal pushing when cervix not fully dilated

Management

Initial

See Figure 43.

Subsequent

- Close monitoring – ? special/intensive care
- Debriefing
- Bereavement care if perinatal death
- Psychological support – especially if hysterectomy
- Consider future pregnancies, e.g. timing, management

Complications

- Severe haemorrhage
- DIC
- Maternal death
  - five between 1994–1996 (Lewis 1998)
  - one between 1997–1999 (Lewis 2001)
  - one between 2000–2002 (Lewis 2004)
  - three between 2003–2005 (Lewis 2007)
- Perinatal death
- Complicated subsequent pregnancies
- Hysterectomy/infertility
- Long-term psychological problems

Student activity

- Note your local policy
- Familiarise yourself with local intensive care charts/records
- Further reading: Kayani and Alfirevic (2005); Kroll and Lyne (2002)

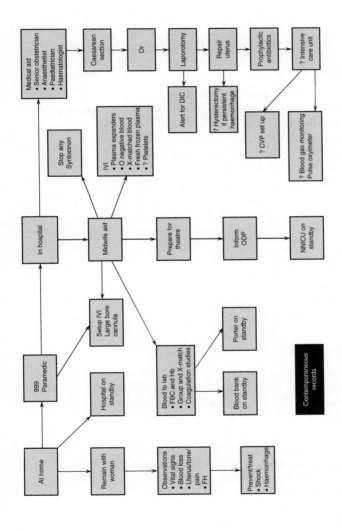

Figure 43 Uterine rupture.

Vaginal examination (VE)

- An intimate procedure that is part of the midwife's role
- May cause distress, discomfort, embarrassment – consider the possible response of survivors of sexual abuse

Indications

- Confirm labour onset/assess progress
- Assess state of membranes/perform ARM (see **Artificial rupture of membranes**)
- Assess fetal position/presentation
- Exclude/diagnose cord prolapse in SRM
- Apply fetal scalp electrode (FSE)
- Confirm full cervical dilatation, i.e. second-stage labour
- Identify second twin's presenting part/perform ARM of second amniotic sac

Aim

- Accurate assessment
- Minimise infection risk
- Maintain woman's dignity/inform of findings
- Keep accurate records

Preparation

- Obtain informed consent
- ? VE pack, ? cleansing solution, ? lubricant, e.g. KY jelly (see note below)
- Sterile gloves
- ? Amnihook if ARM needed
- Partogram to record findings
- Note timing of last VE (commonly 4 hourly)
- Explain procedure/seek consent
- Ensure privacy
- Woman empties bladder
- Perform abdominal palpation

Action

- Woman in dorsal position, knees bent, thighs abducted, relaxed
- Aseptic technique – gloves worn
- ? Vulva swabbed (using left hand, avoiding contamination of examining hand – see Stewart 2005) – note external genitalia
- Two fingers of right hand inserted gently using lubrication
- Assess vaginal condition – is it warm/moist (hot/dry may indicate infection)
- Feel cervix – consistency ? soft/firm; length ? effaced/not; dilatation; application to presenting part
- Feel for forewaters – ? present/absent/bulging; following ARM exclude cord prolapse
- Confirm level of presenting part, i.e. station in relation to pelvic landmarks (see Figure 44)
- Feel for landmarks on fetal skull – determines position
- Note caput formation/moulding
- Assess – ischial spines, ? prominent; angle of pubic arch
- Remove fingers – note show/liquor
- Make woman comfortable/explain findings

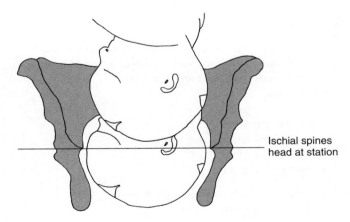

Ischial spines
head at station

Figure 44 Stations of the head in the pelvis.

- Record information accurately (NMC 2009)
- Medical aid prn
- NB: accuracy of findings may only be about 70% (Chou *et al.* 2004; Dupuis *et al.* 2005; Nizard *et al.* 2009)

Student activity

- Note local policies and procedures, e.g. use of a sterile pack, cleansing solution (tap water may be used) and lubricant; the vagina is not strerile but technique should avoid introducing microorganisms
- Further reading: Hobbs (2003); Lewin *et al.* (2005); Stewart (2005); Stuart (2003); Warren (2003)

Varicose veins

See also **Haemorrhoids**.

Enlarged veins commonly in:

- Lower leg
- Vulva
- Anal/rectal area (haemorrhoids)
- Pelvic area

Aetiology

- Weakened valves +/− weak vein walls – poor venous return
- Common antenatally – increased venous stasis caused by:
    (i) gravid uterus raising abdominal pressure
    (ii) large baby
    (iii) multiple pregnancy
    (iv) polyhydramnios
    (v) progesterone relaxing smooth muscle of veins

Signs and symptoms

- Visible superficially as dark blue lines/bulges
- Deep leg/rectal veins not visible

- Aching/heavy sensation
- Oedema
- Local inflammation
- Pain/blood on passing stool (haemorrhoids)

Prevention/management

- Avoid prolonged standing
- Elevate legs/pelvis (NB: supine hypotension)

Legs

Support tights/TED stockings to prevent DVT (see **TED (thrombo-embolic disorder) stockings** and **DVT – deep vein thrombosis** in Section 1)

Vulva

- Thick cotton sanitary pad for support
- Care at delivery

Haemorrhoids

Avoid constipation with high-fibre diet, adequate fluid intake, mild laxative, e.g. Lactulose

Complications

- Increased risk of thrombophlebitis/DVT
- Pain/discomfort
- Ruptured vulval veins/haemorrhage at delivery
- Irritation/bleeding haemorrhoids
- Long-term morbidity – pain/aching, stress about appearance

Student activity

Further reading: Allen (2009).

Venepuncture

Aim

To obtain specimen of venous blood for laboratory tests.

Preparation

Tray with:
• Appropriate colour-coded, correctly labelled vacuumised blood collection sysem, e.g. Vacutainer®; or blood bottles, needle and syringe
• Skin-cleansing swab
• Tourniquet
• Hand hygiene; then ? gloves – personal preference (NB: health and safety)
• Skin plaster/micropore tape
• Sterile cotton wool/gauze swabs
• Laboratory request forms – completed and transport bag
• Biohazard labels if required, e.g. client carrier of Hepatitis B
• Sharps container

Action

• Identify client/explain procedure/seek consent
• Client sitting comfortably
• Support client's preferred arm
• Inspect and palpate veins/determine which is suitable – commonly median basilica in antecubital fossa (at elbow); avoid infusion sites, areas of infection/trauma
• Apply tourniquet on upper arm – maximum duration 2 minutes
• Prepare containers/needle and syringe
• Cleanse area with swab for 30 seconds – allow to dry for 30 seconds
• Insert needle into vein at angle of $15°$–$30°$
• Obtain specimen(s) prn in following order:
  (i) tubes without additives first
  (ii) then coagulation tubes
  (iii) tubes with additives
• Release tourniquet
• Remove needle whilst applying digital pressure with dry cotton wool

- Apply plaster/gauze and micropore tape
- Dispose of equipment safely – do not resheath needle
- Wash hands
- Dispatch to laboratory
- Record in case notes

Student activity

- Education and training required before undertaking
- Note your unit policy for venepuncture – NB: students may be prohibited from performing
- Further reading: Lavery and Ingram (2005); Scales (2008a)

Ventouse delivery

See **Instrumental delivery**.

Vomiting

See **Nausea and vomiting**.

Winterton report (1992)

Parliamentary Select Committee on Health.

Second report on the maternity services. A major report published by the Health Committee of the House of Commons: chair Nicholas Winterton. After a year-long enquiry collecting evidence from mothers and midwives in Sweden, the Netherlands, Belfast, Cardiff, Leeds, Oxford and elsewhere, the report gave recommendations to improve maternity services. Some have been implemented, e.g. that women should be partners in their community-based care, greater professional continuity, promotion of breast-feeding, a paramedic service able to deal with obstetric emergencies and client-held notes. Others, e.g. raising maternity benefits for the young and low-paid, improvement in status, pay and conditions for midwives and trainee status for SHOs under midwives' supervision, have not been accepted. The report led to the setting up of an Expert Maternity Group under Baroness Cumberlege, which resulted in the publication of *Changing Childbirth* by the Department of Health (DH 1993).

References

Allen, L. (2009) Assessment and management of patients with varicose veins. *Nursing Standard* 23(23): 49–57

American Academy of Family Physicians. (2005) *DR C BRAVADO ALSO: Mnemonic Reference Cards*. Online: http://www.aafp.org/also

APEC (1994) *Fact Sheet 1: Low-Dose Aspirin for High-Risk Pregnancy*. Action on Pre-eclampsia (registered charity). Abbots Langley, Herts

Ayers, J.F. (2000) The use of alternative therapies in the support of breastfeeding. *Journal of Human Lactation* 16(1): 52–56

Bailey, N., Brown, G., Di Marco, H., *et al.* (2004) Teenage pregnancy: medical encounters. *British Journal of Midwifery* 12(11): 680–685

Barrett, C., Richens, A. (2002) Epilepsy and pregnancy: report of an epilepsy research foundation workshop. *Epilepsy Research* 522(3): 147–187

Barrowclough, D. (2009) Preparing for pregnancy. Chapter 13. In: *Myles's Textbook for Midwives*, 15th edition. Fraser, D.M., Cooper, M.A. (eds), Edinburgh, Churchill Livingstone Elsevier

Baston, H. (2004a) Perineal repair. *Practising Midwife* 7(9): 12–15

Baston, H. (2004b) Midwifery basics: postnatal care principles. *Practising Midwife* 7(11): 40–45

Bastos, M.H., McCourt, C. (2010) Morbidity during the postnatal period: impact on women and society. Chapter 6. In: *Essential Midwifery Practice: Postnatal Care*, Byrom, S., Edwards, G., Bick, D. (eds), Chichester, Wiley Blackwell

Bauld, L., Bell, K., McCullough, L., Richardson, L., Greaves, L. (2009) The effectiveness of NHS smoking cessation services: a systematic review. *Journal of Public Health* Advanced Access July 28: 1–12. Online: http://www.jpublichealth.oxfordjournals.org (2009). Accessed 20/10/09

Beckmann, M.M., Garrett, A.J. (2006) Antenatal perineal massage for reducing perineal trauma. *Cochrane Database of Systematic Reviews* (1): CD005123

Bewley, S., Shannon, A. (2007) Peer review and the term breech trial. *The Lancet* 569(9565): 906

References

Bick, D. (2010) Contemporary postnatal care in the twenty first century. Chapter 2. In: *Essential Midwifery Practice: Postnatal Care*, Byrom, S., Edwards, G., Bick, D. (eds), Chichester, Wiley Blackwell

Bifulco, A. (2004) Maternal attachment style and depression associated with childbirth: preliminary results from a European and US cross-cultural study. *British Journal of Psychiatry* 184: s31–s37

Bø, K., Owe, K.M., Nystad, W., (2007) Which women do pelvic floor muscle exercises 6 months' postpartum? *American Journal of Obstetrics and Gynecology* 197: 49.e1–49.e5

Boulvain, M., Stan, C., Irion, O. (2005) Membrane sweeping for induction of labour. *The Cochrane Database of Systemic Reviews* (1): CD000451. DOI: 10.1002/14651858.CD000451.pub2

Boyle, M. (2002) *Emergencies Around Childbirth*. Radcliffe Medical Press, Abingdon, Oxon

Briscoe, L., Clark, S., Yoxall, C.W. (2002) Can transcutaneous billirubinometry reduce the need for blood tests in jaundiced full term babies? *Archives of Diseases of Childhood. Fetal and Neonatal Edition* 83(3): F190–F192

Brownlee, K., Oikonen, J. (2004) Towards a theoretical framework for perinatal bereavement. *British Journal of Social Work* 34: 517–529

Bushell, A., McNinch, A., Tripp, J. (2007) Neonatal Vitamin K prophylaxis in great Britain and Ireland: the impact of perceived risk and product licensing effectiveness. *Archives of Disease and Childhood* 92: 754–758

Callister, L.C. (2006) Perinatal loss: a family perspective. *Journal of Perinatal and Neonatal Nursing* 20(3): 227–236

Carroli, G., Migninil, L. (2009) Episiotomy for vaginal birth. *Cochrane Database of Systematic Reviews* (1): CD00081

Cedergren, M.I. (2007) Optimal gestation weight gain for BMI categories. *Obstetrics and Gynecology* 110(4): 759–764

CEMACH (2008) *Perinatal mortality 2006: England, Wales and Northern Ireland*. CEMACH, London

Chen, X.-K., Wen, S.W., Flemming, N., Demissie, K., Rhoads, G.G. (2007) Teenage pregnancy and adverse birth outcomes: a large population based retrospective study. *International Journal of Epidemiology* 36(2): 368–373

Chou, M., Kreiser, D., Taslimi, M., Druzin, M., El-Sayed, Y. (2004) Vaginal versus ultrasound examination of fetal occiput position during the second stage of labor. *American Journal of Obstetrics and Gynecology* 191(2): 521–524

Clarkson, L.J. (2001) Retinopathy of prematurity: Part 1. A fresh look at its cause. *Journal of Neonatal Nursing* 7(6): 186–189

Clarkson, L.J. (2002) Retinopathy of prematurity: Part 2. Current treatment options. *Journal of Neonatal Nursing* 8(1): 7–10

Clutton-Brock, T. (2007) Critical care. Chapter 19 & Annex A. In: *The Confidential Enquiry into Maternal and Child Health (CEMACH). Saving Mothers' Lives: Reviewing Maternal Deaths to Make Motherhood Safer – 2003–2005*, The Seventh Report on Confidential Enquiries into Maternal Deaths in the UK, Lewis, G. (ed.), London, CEMACH

Connolly, G., Naidoo, C., Conroy, R.M., Byrne, P., McKenna, P. (2003) A new predictor of cephalo-pelvic disproportion. *Journal of Obstetrics and Gynaecology* 23(1): 27–29

Coombes, J. (2000) Cholestasis in pregnancy: a challenging disorder. *British Journal of Midwifery* 8(9): 565–570

Couch, S.C., Deckelbaum, R.J. (2008) Obesity and pregnancy. Chapter 5. In: *Nutrition and Health: Handbook of Nutrition and Pregnancy*. Lammie-Keefe, C.J., Couch, S.C., Philipson, C.E. (eds), Totowa, NJ, Humana Press

Crafter, H. (2009) Problems in pregnancy. Chapter 20. In: *Myles's Textbook for Midwives*, 15th edition, Fraser, D.M., Cooper, M.A., (eds), Edinburgh, Churchill Livingstone Elsevier

Currid, T. (2004) Clinical issues relating to puerperal psychosis and its management. *Nursing Times* 100(17): 40–43

Currie, L., Morrell, C., Scrivener, R. (2003) *Clinical Governance: An RCN Resource Guide*. Royal College of Nursing. Online: http://www.rcn.org.uk

Dahlen, H.G., Homer, C.S.E. (2008) What the views of midwives in relation to perineal suturing? *Women and Birth* 21(1): 27–35

Davies, B.R. (2003) Early detection and treatment of postnatal depression in primary care. *Journal of Advanced Nursing* 44(3): 248–255

Dcsf (Department for Children, Schools & Families). (2003) *Every Child Matters*. Online: http://www.dcsf.gov.uk

Dcsf (Department for Children, Schools & Families). (2006) *Working Together to Safeguard Children: A Guide to Inter-agency Working to Safeguard and Promote the Welfare of Children*. Online: http://www.dcsf.gov.uk

Dcsf (Department for Children, Schools & Families). (2007) *Teenage Pregnancy*. Online: http://www.dcsf.gov.uk

Deane-Gray, T. (2004) Education for parenthood. Chapter 22. In: *Mayes' Midwifery*, 13th edition, Henderson, C., Macdonald, S. (eds), Edinburgh, Ballière Tindall

Deken, A. (2008) Neonatal jaundice: implications for newborn health. Chapter 13. In: *Examination of Newborn and Neonatal Health: A Multidimensional Approach*. Davies, L., McDonald, S. (eds), Philadelphia, Churchill Livingstone Elsevier

Demott, K., Bick, D., Norman, R., *et al.* (2006) *Clinical Guidelines and Evidence for Postnatal Care: Routing Postnatal Care of Recently Delivered Women and Their*

References

Babies. National Collaborating Centre for Primary Care and the Royal College of General Practitioners, London. Online: http://www.nice.org.uk/CG37

DH (Department of Health). (1993) *Changing Childbirth. Report of the Expert Maternity Group*. HMSO, London

DH (Department of Health). (1997) *The New NHS – Modern, Dependable*. Department of Health, London

DH (Department of Health). (2004) *National Service Framework for Children, Young People and Maternity Services: Maternity Services*. Department of Health. Online: http://www.dh.gov.uk

DH. (2007a) *Maternity Matters: Choice, Access and Continuity of Care in a Safe Service*. Department of Health. Online: http://www.dh.gov.uk

DH. (2007b) *Implementation Plan for Reducing Health Inequalities in Infant Mortality: A Good Practice Guide*. Department of Health, Health Inequalities Unit. Online: http://www.dh.gov.uk

Dimond, B. (2006) *Legal Aspects of Midwifery*, 3rd edition, Cheshire, Books for Midwives

Dougherty, L. (2008a) Intravenous therapy: recognising the difference between infiltration and extravasation. *British Journal of Nursing* 17(14): 896,898–901

Dougherty, L. (2008b) Peripheral cannulation. *Nursing Standard* 22(52): 49–56

Dowswell, T., Neilson, J.P. (2009) Intervention for heartburn in pregnancy. *Cochrane Database of Systematic Reviews* Oct. 8 (4): CD007065

Draycott, T., Broad, G., Chidley, K. (2000) The development of an eclampsia box and 'fire drill'. *British Journal of Midwifery* 8(1): 26–30

Drife, J. (2007) Thrombosis and thromboembolism, Chapter 2. In: *Saving Mothers Lives*. Lewis, G. (ed.), The seventh confidential enquiry into maternal deaths in the UK 2003–2005, London, CEMACH

Dryden, C., Young, D., Hepburn, M., Mactier, H. (2009) Maternal methadone use in pregnancy: factors associated with the development of neonatal abstinence syndrome and implications for health care resources. *British Journal of Obstetrics and Gynaecology* 116(5): 665–671

Dubowitz, L.M.S., Dubowitz, V., Goldberg, B.A.C. (1970) Clinical assessment of gestational age in the newborn infant. *The Journal of Pediatrics* 77(1): 1.10

Dubowitz, L., Mercuri, E., Dubowitz, V. (1998) An optimality score for the neurologic examination of the term newborn. *The Journal of Pediatrics* 133(3): 406–416

Duckitt, K., Harrington, D. (2005) Risk factors for pre-eclampsia at antenatal booking: systematic review of controlled studies. *British Medical Journal* 330: 565

Duley, L., Gülmezoglu, A.M., Henderson-Smart, D.J. (2003) Magnesium sulphate and other anticonvulsants for women with pre-eclampsia. *The Cochrane Database of Systematic Reviews* (2): Art. No. CD000025. DOI: 10.1002/14651858.CD000025

Duley, L., Henderson-Smart, D.J., Meher, S., King, J.F., (2007) Antiplatelet agents for preventing pre-eclampsia and its complications. *Cohocrane Database of Systematic Reviews* (2): Art. No.: CD004659. DOI: 10.1002/14651858. CD004659. pub2

Duley, L., Watkins, K. (1999) The Magpie trial: magnesium sulphate for pre-eclampsia. *British Journal of Midwifery* 7(10): 617–619

Dupuis, O., Ruimark, S., Corinne, D., Simone, T., Andrė, D., Renė-Charles, R. (2005) Fetal head position during the second stage of labour: comparison of digital vaginal examination and transabdominal ultrasonographic examination. *European Journal of Obstetrics and Gynecology and Reproductive Biology* 123(2): 193–197

Ebert, L.M., Freeman, L., Fahy, K., van der Riet, P. (2009) Midwives interaction with women who smoke in pregnancy. *British Journal of Midwifery* 17(1): 24–29

Edwards, G., Gordon, U., Atherton, J. (2005) Network approach boosts midwives' public health role. *British Journal of Midwifery* 13(1): 48–53

Every, M. (1994) Meeting Report: CLASP trial. *Midwives Chronicle and Nursing Notes* 107(1281): 402

Farnell, S., Maxwell, L., Tan, S., Rhodes, A., Philips, B. (2005) Temperature measurement: comparison of non-invasive methods used in adult critical care. *Journal of Clinical Nursing* 14(5): 632–639

Feig, D.S., Palda, V.A. (2002) Type 2 diabetes in pregnancy – a growing concern. *The Lancet* 359(9318): 520–525

Finigan, V., Davies, S. (2004) 'I just wanted to love, hold him forever': women's lived experience of skin-to-skin contact with their baby immediately after birth. *Evidence Based Midwifery* 2(2): 59–65

Fletcher, J., Ball, G. (2006) Chlamydia screening in pregnancy: a missed opportunity? *British Journal of Midwifery* 14(7): 390–392

Food Standards Agency. (2007) *Folic Acid Fortification*. Online: http://www.food. gov.uk Accessed 7/11/09

Fraser, D., Mukhopadhyay, S., (2009) Nutrition and hydration in labour. In: *Best Practice in Labour and Delivery*. Warren, R., Arulkumaran, S. (eds), Cambridge, Cambridge University Press

FSID (Foundation for the Study of Infant Death). (2009) *Cot Death Fact and Figures*. Online: http://www.fsid.org. Accessed 19.10.09

References

Gardosi, J., Francis, A. (1999) Controlled trial of fundal height measurement plotted on customised antenatal growth charts. *British Journal of Obstetrics and Gynaecology* 106: 309–317

Gibbon, K. (2004) Developments in perinatal mental health assessments. *British Journal of Midwifery* 12(12): 754–760

Gibson, J. (2008) How to perform an abdominal palpation. *Midwives* 11(5): 22

Glazerman, M. (2006) Five years of the Term Breech Trial: the rise and fall of a randomized controlled trial. *American Journal of Obstetrics and Gynecology* 194(1): 20–25

Glueck, C.J., Wang, P., Kobayashi, S., Phillips, H., Steve-Smith, L. (2002) Metformin therapy throughout pregnancy reduces the development of gestational diabetes in women with polycystic ovary syndrome. *Fertility and Sterility: The Official Journal of the American Society for Reproductive Medicine* 77(3): 520–529

Goldenberg, R., Culhae, J., Iams, J., Romero, R. (2008) Epidemiology and causes of preterm birth. *The Lancet* 371(9606): 75–84

Greenes, V., Williamson, C. (2009) Intra-hepatic cholestasis of pregnancy. *World Journal of Gastroenterology* 15(7): 2049–2066

Guerewitsch, E.D., Kim, E.J., Yang, J.H., *et al.* (2005) Comparing McRobert's and Rubin's maneuvers for initial managment of shoulder dystocia: an objective evaluation. *American Journal of Obstetric and Gynecology* 192(1): 153–160

Handley, A. (2005) *Adult Basic Life Support. Resuscitation Council (UK) Guidelines.* Online: http://www.resus.org.uk

Hannah, M.E., Hannah, W.J., Hewson, S.A. (2000) Planned caesarean section versus planned vaginal birth for breech presentation at term: a randomised multicentre trial. *The Lancet* 356: 1375–1383

Harris, J. (2009) How to take a mother's temperature. *Midwives: The Official Magazine of the RCM* Oct/Nov.: 27

Hart, E.S., Grottkay, B.E., Rebells, G.E., Albright, M.B. (2005) The newborn foot: diagnosis and management of common conditions. *Orthopaedic Nursing* 24(5): 313–321

Hay-Smith, J., Mørkved, S., Fairbrother, K.A., Herbison, G.P. (2008) Pelvic floor muscle training for prevention and treatment of urinary and faecal incontinence in antenatal and postnatal women. *Cochrane Database Systematic Review* Oct. 8(4): CD007471

Heath, P.T., Balfour, G.F., Tighe, H., Verlander, N.Q., Lamaagni, T.L., Efstratiou, A. (2009) Group B streptococcal disease in infants: a case control study. *Archives of Disease in Childhood* 94(9): 674–680

Henderson, J.J., Evans, S.F., Straton, J.A.Y., *et al.* (2003) Impact of postnatal depression on breastfeeding duration. *Birth* 30(3): 175–180

Hendrick, V. (2003) Treatment of postnatal depression: effective interventions are available, but the condition remains under diagnosed. *British Medical Journal* 327(7422): 1003–1004

Hernández-Diáz, S., Toh, S., Cnattingius, S. (2009) Risk of pre-eclampsia in first and subsequent pregnancies: prospective cohort study. *British Medical Journal* 338: b2255

Heslehurst, N., Lang, R., Rankin, J., Wilkinson, J.R., Summerbell, C.D. (2007) Obesity in pregnancy: a study of the impact of maternal obesity on NHS maternity services. *British Journal of Obstetrics and Gynaecology* 114: 334–342

Hey, E. (2003) Vitamin K – what, why and when. *Archives of Disease in Childhood – Fetal and Neonatal* 88: 80–83

Hicks, C., Spurgeon, P., Barwell, F. (2003) Changing childbirth: a pilot project. *The Journal of Advanced Nursing* 42 (6): 617–628

Higgins, J.R., de Swiet, M. (2001) Blood pressure measurement and classification in pregnancy. *The Lancet* 357(9250): 131–135

Hildingsson, I., Radestad, I., Rubertsson, C. (2003) Few women wish to be delivered by caesarean section. *Obstetric and Gynecological Survey* 58(1): 15–16

Hillier, D. (2003) *Childbirth in the Global Village: Implications for Midwifery Education and Practice*. Routledge Taylor- Francis Group, London

Hobbs, L. (2003) Assessing cervical dilatation without VEs: watching the purple line. In: *Midwifery Best Practice*. Wickham, S. (ed.), Edinburgh, Books for Midwives Press

Hunter, S., Hofmeyr, G.J., Kulier, R. (2007) Hands and knees position in late pregnancy or labour for fetal malposition (lateral or posterior). *Cochrane Database of Systematic Reviews* (4): CD001063

Ingram, P., Lavery, I. (2007) Peripheral intravenous cannulation: safe insertion and removal technique. *Nursing Standard* 22(1): 44–48

Jansson, L.M., Choo, R.E., Harrow, C., *et al.* (2007) Concentration of methadone in breast milk and plasma in the immediate postnatal period. *Journal of Human Lactation* 23(2): 184–190

Jones, C.A., Walker, K.S., Badawi, N. (2009) Antiviral agents for treatment of herpes simplex virus infection in neonates. *Cochrane Database of Systematic Reviews* (3): CD004206

Kayani, S.I., Alfirevic, Z. (2005) Uterine rupture after induction of labour in women with previous caesarean section. *British Journal of Obstetrics and Gynaecology* 112(4): 451–453

Kennedy, H.P., MacDonald, E.L. (2002) 'Altered consciousness' during childbirth: potential clues to post traumatic stress disorder? *Journal of Midwifery and Women's Health* 47(5): 380–382

References

Kenyon, S. (1995) ORACLE – an overview of the evidence. *MIDIRS Midwifery Digest* 5(1): 14–16

Kenyon, S., Boulvain, M., Neilson, J. (2004) Antibiotics for preterm rupture of the membranes: a systematic review. *Obstetrics Gynecology* 104(5 part 1): 1051–1057

Kenyon, S., Taylor, D.J. (2002) The effects of the publication of a major clinical trial in a high impact journal on clinical practice: the ORACLE trial experience. *British Journal of Obstetrics and Gynaecology* 109(12): 1341–1343

Keren, R., Tremont, K., Luan, X., Cnaan, A. (2009) Visual assessment of jaundice in term and late preterm infants. *Archives of Diseases of Childhood – Fetal and Neonatal Edition* 94(5): F317–F322

Kettle, C., Hills, R.K., Ismail, K.M. (2007) Continuous versus interrupted suture for repair of episiotomy and second degree tears. *Cochrane Database of Systematic Reviews* (4): CD000947

Kettle, C., Hills, R., Jones, P., Darby, L., Gray, R., Johanson, R. (2002) Continuous versus interrupted perineal repair with rapidly absorbed sutures after spontaneous vaginal birth: a randomised controlled trial. *The Lancet* 359(9325): 2217–2223

Kidger, J. (2004) Including young mothers: limitations to New Labour's strategy for supporting teenage parents. *Critical Social Policy* 24(3): 291–311

Kightley, R. (2008) Postnatal depression and unhappiness. *British Journal of Midwifery* 16(4): 258–260

King, J., Flenady, V. (2002) Prophylactic antibiotics for inhibiting preterm labour with intact membranes. *The Cochrane Database of Systemic Reviews* (4): CD000246 Accessed 15/02/05

Kroll, D., Lyne, M. (2002) Chapter 8: Uterine inversion and uterine rupture. In: *Emergencies Around Childbirth: A Handbook for Midwives*. Boyle, M. (ed.), Abingdon, Oxon, Radcliffe Medical Press

Labiner-Wolf, J., Fein, S.B., Shealy, K., Wang, C. (2008) Prevalence of breast milk expression and associated factors. *Pediatrics* 122 (Suppl. 2): S63–S68

Lacasse, A., Rey, E., Ferreira, E., Morin, C., Bérand, A. (2009) Determinants of early medical management of nausea and vomiting of pregnancy. *Birth: Issues in Perinatal Care* 36(1): 70–77

Lachelin, G.C.S., McGarrigie, H.H.G., Seed, P.T., Brieley, A., Shennan, A.H., Poston, L. (2009) Low saliva progesterone concentrations are associated with spontaneous early preterm labour (before 34 weeks of gestation) in women at increased risk of preterm delivery. *British Journal of Obstetrics and Gynaecology* 116(11): 1515–1519

Laing, K.G. (2001) Post-traumatic stress disorder: myth or reality? *British Journal of Midwifery* 9(7): 447–452

Langley, V., Thoburn, A., Shaw, S., Barton, A. (2006) Second degree tears: to suture or not? A randomised controlled trial. *British Journal of Midwifery* 14(9): 550–554

Lavender, T., Hart, A., Smyth, R.M. (2008) Effects of program use on outcomes for women in spontaneous labour at term. *Cochrane Database of Systematic Reviews* CD005461

Lavery, I., Ingram, P. (2005) Venepuncture: best practice. *Nursing Standard* 19(49): 55–65

Layton, S. (2004) The effects of perineal trauma on women's health. *British Journal of Midwifery* 12(4): 231–236

Levi, M. (2009) Disseminated Intravascular Coagulation (DIC) in pregnancy and the peripartum period. *Thrombosis Research* 23(2): s63–s64

Lewin, D., Fearon, B., Hemmings, V., Johnson, G. (2005) Informing women during vaginal examination. *British Journal of Midwifery* 13(1): 26–29

Lewis, G. (ed.) (1998) *Why Mothers Die. 1994–1996. Report on the Confidential Enquiries into Maternal Deaths in the United Kingdom.* HMSO, London

Lewis, G. (ed.) (2001) *Why Mothers Die 1997–1999. Report on the Confidential Enquiries into Maternal Deaths in the United Kingdom.* London, RCOG Press

Lewis, G. (ed.) (2004) *Why Mothers Die 2000–2002 Confidential Enquiry into Maternal and Child Health.* London, RCOG Press

Lewis, G. (ed.) (2007) The Confidential Enquiry into Maternal and Child Health (CEMACH). *Saving Mothers' Lives: Reviewing Maternal Deaths to Make Motherhood Safer – 2003–2005.* The Seventh Report on Confidential Enquiries into Maternal Deaths in the UK. London, CEMACH

Lilford, R.J., Van Coeverden de Groot, H.A., Moore, P.J., Bingham, P. (2005) The relative risks of caesarean section (intrapartum or elective) and vaginal delivery: a detailed analysis to exclude the effects of medical disorders and other acute pre-existing physiological disturbances. *British Journal of Obstetrics and Gynaecology. An International Journal of Obstetrics and Gynaecology* 97(10): 883–892,463

Lim, J.Y., Arulkumaran, S. (2008) Meconium aspiration syndrome. *Obstetrics, Gynaecology and Reproductive Medicine* 18(4): 106–109

Lindsay, P. (2004) Preterm labour. Chapter 50. In: *Mayes' Midwifery*, 13th edition, Henderson, C., Macdonald, S., Edinburgh, Ballière Tindall

Liston, W. (2007) Haemorrhage. Chapter 4. In: *The Confidential Enquiry into Maternal and Child Health (CEMACH) Saving Mothers' Lives: Reviewing Maternal Deaths to Make Motherhood Safer – 2003–2005.* The Seventh Report on Confidential Enquiries into Maternal Deaths in the UK. Lewis, G. (ed.), London, CEMACH

References

Lorente, C., Cordier, S., Goujard, J., *et al.* (2000) Tobacco and alcohol use during pregnancy and risk of oral clefts. *American Journal of Public Health* 90(3): 415–419

McAllion, D. (2004) Fundal height and low birth weight. *British Journal of Midwifery* 12(2): 101–104

McCandlish, R. (1999) The HOOP study: a personal view. *MIDIRS Midwifery Digest* 9(1): 77–78

McCandlish, R. (2001) Perineal trauma: prevention and treatment. *Journal of Midwifery and Women's Health* 46(6): 396–401

McCandlish, R., Bowler, U., Van Hasten, H., *et al.* (1998) A randomised controlled trial of care of the perineum during second stage of normal labour. *British Journal of Obstetrics and Gynaecology* 105(12): 1262–1272

Abstract in (1999) *MIDIRS Midwifery Digest* 9(1): 76

McCowan, L.M.E., Dekker, G.A., Chan, E., *et al.* (2009) Spontaneous preterm birth and small for gestational age infants in women who stop smoking early in pregnancy: prospective cohort study. *British Medical Journal* 338: b1081

McDonald, S.J., Middleton, P. (2008) Effects of timing of umbilical cord clamping of term infants on maternal and neonatal outcomes (Review). *The Cochrane Collaboration* (2): Art. No. CD004074

McKay-Moffat, S. (ed.) (2007) *Disability in Pregnancy and Childbirth.* Edinburgh, Churchill Livingstone Elsevier

McParlin, C., Graham, R.H., Robson, S.C. (2008) Caring for women with nausea and vomiting in pregnancy: new approaches. *British Journal of Midwifery* 16(5): 280–285

Magann, E.F., Isler, C.M., Chauhan, S.P., Martin, J.N. (2000) Amniotic fluid volume estimation and the biophysical profile: a confusion of criteria. *Obstetrics and Gynecology* 96(4): 640–642

Mahran, M.A., Sayed, A.T., Imoh-Ita, F. (2008) Avoiding over diagnosis of shoulder dystocia. *Journal of Obstetrics and Gynaecology* 28(2): 173–176

Mains, J.A., Coxall, K., Lloyd, H. (2008) Measuring temperature. *Nursing Standard* 22(39): 44–47

Maisels, M., Watchko, J. (2003) Treatment of jaundice in low birth weight infants. *Archives of Diseases in Childhood: Fetal and Neonatal Edition* 88(6): F459–F463

Mantle, F. (2001) The role of alternative medicine in treating postnatal depression. *British Journal of Community Nursing* 6(7): 363–368

Metcalf, A., Bick, D., Tohill, S., Williams, A., Haldon, V. (2006) A prospective cohort study of repair and non-repair of second degree perineal trauma: results and issues for future research. *Evidence Based Midwifery* 4(2): 60–64

Meyer, M., Wagner, K., Bennenuto, A., Plante, D., Howard, D. (2007) Intrapartum and postpartum analgesia for women maintained on methadone during pregnancy. *Obstetrics and Gynecology* 110(2): 261–266

Miller, J., Turan, S., Baschat, A. (2008) Fetal growth restriction. *Seminars in Perinatology* 32(4): 274–280

Mills, J.E., Tudehope, D. (2001) Fibreoptic phototherapy for neonatal jaundice. *The Cochrane Library* (1): Ant. No. CD002060. DOI: 10.1002/14651858.CD.002060

Misuse of Drug Regulations (2001) http://www.homeoffice.gov.uk

Modder, J. (ed.) (2009) The Confidential Enquiry into Maternal and Child Health (CEMACH). *Perinatal Mortality 2007. The Fifth Report on Perinatal Mortality.* London, CEMACH

Moon, R.Y., Horne, R.S.C., Hauck, F.R. (2007) Sudden infant death syndrome. *The Lancet* 370(9598): 1578–1587

Morley, A. (2004) Pre-eclampsia: pathophysiology and its management. *British Journal of Midwifery* 12(1): 30–31, 34–37

Morris, W., Tay, K.K. (2008) Strategies for preventing peripheral intravenous cannula infection. *British Journal of Nursing* (IV Therapy Supplement) 17(19): S14–S21

Moyzakitis, W. (2004) Exploring women's descriptions of distress and/or trauma in childbirth from a feminist perspective. *Evidence Based Midwifery* 2(1): 8–14

Muramoto, O. (2001) Bioethical aspects of the recent changes in the policy of refusal of blood by Jehova's Witnesses. *British Medical Journal* 322: 37–39

Murphy, D.J., MacKenzie, I.Z. (2005) The mortality and morbidity associated with umbilical cord prolapse. *British Journal of Obstetrics and Gynaecology* 102(10): 826–830

National Research Council & Institute of Medicine (2007) *Influences of Pregnancy Weight Gain on Maternal and Child Health: A Workshop.* Chapter 2. Trends in maternal and gestational weight. Washington, DC, National Academies Press

Naughten, F. (2005) The heel prick: how efficient is common practice? *Midwives* 8(3): 112–114

Neilson, J. (2007) Pre-eclampsia and eclampsia. In: Lewis, G. (ed.), *The Confidential Enquiry into Maternal and Child Health (CEMACH) Saving Mothers' Lives: Reviewing Maternal Deaths to Make Motherhood Safer – 2003–2005. The Seventh Report on Confidential Enquiries into Maternal Deaths in the UK.* London, CEMACH

Nevi, I., Aiorla, G., Contu, G., Allais, G., Facchinetti, F., Benedetto, C. (2004) Acupuncture plus moxibustion to resolve breech presentation: a randomized controlled study. *The Journal of Maternal-Fetal and Neonatal Medicine* 15: 247–252

References

NICE. (2006) *Therapeutic Amnioinfusion for Oligohydramnios during Pregnancy (Excluding Labour): Intervention Guideline 192*. National Institute for Health and Clinical Excellence. Online: http://www.nice.org.uk

NICE. (2007) *Intrapartum Care: Care of Healthy Women and Their Babies during Childbirth*. National Institute for Health and Clinical Excellence. Online: http://www.nice.org.uk

NICE. (2008a) *Antenatal Care: Routine Care for Pregnant Woman. Clinical Guideline 62*. National Institute for Health and Clinical Excellence. Online: http://www.nice.org.uk

NICE. (2008b) *Improving the Nutrition of Pregnancy and Breastfeeding Mothers and Children in Low-income Households. Public Health Guideline 11*. National Institute for Health and Clinical Excellence. Online: http://www.nice.org.uk

NICE. (2008c) *Induction of Labour. Clinical Guideline 70*. National Institute for Health and Clinical Excellence. Online: http://www.nice.org.uk

NICE. (2008d) *Diabetes in Pregnancy: Management of Diabetes and Its Complications from Pre-conception to the Postnatal Period. Clinical Guideline 63*. National Institute for Health and Clinical Excellence. Online: http://www.nice.org.uk

Nizard, J., Haberman, S., Paltieli, R., *et al.* (2009) How reliable is the determination of cervical dilatation? Comparison of vaginal examination with spatial position-tracking ruler. *American Journal of Obstetrics and Gynecology* 200(4): 402.e1–402.e4

NMC. (2004) *Midwives' Rules and Standards*. London, Nursing and Midwifery Council

NMC. (2007) *Standards for Medicines Management*. London, Nursing and Midwifery Council

NMC. (2008) *Standards of Conduct, Performance and Ethics for Nurses and Midwives* (The Code). London, Nursing and Midwifery Council

NMC. (2009) *Record Keeping: Guidance for Nurses and Midwives*. London, Nurses and Midwives Council

Norman, P., Gregory, I., Dorling, D., Baker, A. (2008) *Geographical Trends in Infant Mortality in England and Wales 1970–2006*. Office for National Statistics. Online: http://www.statistics.gov.uk

Nursing and Midwifery Order. (2001) *Statutory Instruments*. Online: http://www.opsi.gov.uk

O'Leary, J.A. (2008) *Shoulder Dystocia and Birth Injury. Prevention and Treatment*. Totana, USA, Humana Press

Office for National Statistics (ONS) (2010) *Statistical Bulletin: Childhood, Infant and Perinatal Mortality in England and Wales, 2008*. Online: http://www.ons.gov.uk

Ohlsson, A., Shah, V.S. (2009) Intrapartum antibiotics for known group B streptococcal colonization. *Cochrane Database of Systematic Reviews* (3): CD007467

Olsen, O. (1999) Expected date of delivery. *British Journal of Obstetrics and Gynaecology* 106(9): 1000

Osadchy, A., Kasmin, A., Koren, G. (2009) Nicotine replacement therapy during pregnancy: recommended or not recommended. *Journal of Obstetric Gynaecology Canada* 31(80): 744–747

Paranjothy, S., Broughton, H., Adappa, R., Fone, D. (2009) Teenage pregnancy: who suffers? *Archive of Diseases of Childhood* 94(3): 239–245

Platt, M.J., Stanistreet, M., Cxasson, F., *et al.* (2002) St Vincent's declaration 10 years on: outcomes of diabetic pregnancies. *Diabetic Medicine* 19(3): 216–220

Premkumar, G. (2005) Perineal trauma: reducing associated postnatal maternal morbidity. *Midwives* 8(1): 30–32

Pritchard, M.A., Beller, E.M., Norton, B. (2005) Skin exposure during conventional phototherapy in preterm infants: a randomized controlled trial. *NNIC* 18(2): 25–27

Quijano, C.E., Abalos, E. (2005) Conservative management of symptomatic and/or complicated haemorrhoids in pregnancy and the puerperium. *Cochrane Database of Systematic Reviews* (3). Art. No.: CD004077. DOI: 10.1002/14651858.CD004077.pub2.

RCOG (Royal College of Obstetricians & Gynaecologists). (2002) *Green Top Guideline 1B Tocolytic Drugs for Women in Preterm Labour*. RCOG Online: http://www.rcog.org.uk

RCOG (Royal College of Obstetricians & Gynaecologists). (2004) *Green Top Guideline 7 Antenatal Corticosteroids to Prevent Respiratory Distress Syndrome*. RCOG Online: http://www.rcog.org.uk

RCOG (Royal College of Obstetricians & Gynaecologists). (2005) *Green Top Guideline 42 Shoulder Dystocia*. RCOG Online: http://www.rcog.org.uk

RCOG (Royal College of Obstetricians & Gynaecologists). (2007) *A Difficult Birth: What Is Shoulder Dystocia? Information for You*. RCOG Online: http://www.rcog.org.uk

Reder, P., Duncan, S. (2003) Understanding communication in child protection networks. *Child Abuse Review* 2(2): 82–100

Renfrew, M.J., McLoughlin, M., McFadden, A. (2008) Cleaning and Sterilization of infant feeding equipment: a systematic review. *Public health Nutrition* 11: 1188–1199

Rennie, J.M., Sehgal, A., De, A., Kendall, G.S., Cole, T.J. (2009) Range of UK practices regarding thresholds for phototherapy and exchange transfusion in neonatal hypobilirubinaemia. *Archives of Disease of Childhood – Fetal and Neonatal Edition* 94(5): F314–F317

Rumbold, A., Duley, L., Crowther, C.A., Haslam, R.R. (2008) Antioxidants for preventing pre-eclampsia. *Chochrane Database of Systematic Reviews* (1) Art. No.: CD004227. DOI: 10.1002/14651858. CD004227.pub3

References

Sadler, L., Davison, T., McCowan, M. (2001) Maternal satisfaction with active management of labour: a randomized controlled trial. *BIRTH* 28(4): 225–235

Saigal, S., Doyle, L. (2008) An overview of mortality and sequelae of preterm birth from infancy to adulthood. *The Lancet* 371(9608): 261–269

Scales, K. (2008a) A practical guide to venepuncture and blood sampling. *Nursing Standard* 22(29): 29–36

Scales, K. (2008b) Intravenous therapy: a guide to good practice. *British Journal of Nursing* (IV Therapy Supplement) 17(19): S4–S12

Schott, J., Henley, A. (2007) Pregnancy loss and death of a baby: the new Sands Guidelines 2007. *British Journal of Midwifery* 15(4): 195–198

Shakespeare, D. (2004) Exploring midwives' attitudes to teenage pregnancy. *British Journal of Midwifery* 12(5): 320–326, 329

Sibai, B.M. (2004a) Diagnosis, controversies and management of the syndrome of hemolysis, elevated liver enzymes, and low platelet count. *Obstetrics and Gynecology* 103(5 part 1): 981–991

Sibai, B.M. (2004b) Magnesium sulphate prophylaxis in pre-eclampsia: lessons learned from recent trials. *American Journal of Obstetrics and Gynecology* 190(6): 1520–1526

Sibai, B.M. (2005) Diagnosis, prevention and management of eclampsia. *Obstetrics and Gynecology* 105(2): 402–410

Siderov, J. (2008) The newborn eye: visual function and screening for ocular disorders. Chapter 11. In: *Examination of the Newborn and Neonatal Health*. Davis, L., McDonald, S. (eds) Edinburgh, Churchill Livingstone Elsevier

Skotko, B. (2002) Mothers of children with Downs Syndrome reflect on their postnatal support. *Pediatrics* 115(1): 64–67

Smith, G.C.S., Bell, J.P., Bobbie, R. (2003) Caesarean section and risk of unexplained stillbirth in subsequent pregnancy. *The Lancet* 362(9398): 1779–1784

Smith, N., Nolan, M.L. (2009) Antenatal education: principles and practice. Chapter 15. In: *Myles' Textbook for Midwives*, 15th edition, Fraser, D.M., Cooper, M.A. (eds), Edinburgh, Churchill Livingstone Elsevier

Squire, C. (2002) Chapter 9: Shoulder dystocia and umbilical cord prolapse. In: *Emergencies Around Childbirth: A Handbook for Midwives*. Boyle, M. (ed.), Abingdon, Oxon, Radcliffe Medical Press

Steen, M., Marchant, P. (2007) Ice packs and cooling gel pads versus non localized treatment for relief of perineal pain: a randomized controlled trial. *Evidence Based Midwifery* 5(1): 16–22

Stevens, T.P., Blennow, M., Soll, R.F. (2005) Early surfactant administration with brief ventilation vs selective surfactant and continued mechanical ventilation for preterm infants with or at risk for respiratory distress syndrome. *The Cochrane Library* (Oxford) (3): ID#CD003063

Stewart, M. (2005) 'I'm just going to wash you down': sanitizing the vaginal examination. *Journal of Advanced Nursing* 51(6): 587–594

Stuart, C.C. (2003) Invasive actions in labour: where have all the 'old tricks' gone? In: *Midwifery Best Practice*. Wickham, S. (ed.), Edinburgh, Books for Midwives Press

Sultan, A.H., Kettle, C. (2007) Diagnosis of perineal trauma. Chapter 2. In: *Perineal and Anal Sphincter Trauma*. Sultan, A.H., Thakar, R., Fenner, D.E. (eds), London, Springer

Sumner, V. (2002) Underinformed on puerperal psychosis, antenatal and postnatal depression: where are we now and where should we be going? *Community Practitioner* 75(8): 316

Svensson, J., Barclay, L. (2009) Randomized-controlled trial of two antenatal education programmes. *Midwifery* 25(2): 114–125

Sweet, L. (2008) Expressed milk as "connection" and its influence on the construction of motherhood for mothers of preterm infants: a qualitative study. *International Breastfeeding Journal* 3: 30

Thakar, R., Sultan, A.H. (2009) Episiotomy and obstetric perineal trauma. Chapter 17. In: *Best Practice in Labour and Delivery*. Warren, R., Arulkumaran, S. (eds), Cambridge, Cambridge University Press

Thompson, J. (2004) Health problems of women following childbirth: part one. *Community Practitioner* 77(7): 267

Tiran, D., Mack, S. (eds) (2000) *Complementary Therapies for Pregnancy and Childbirth*, 2nd edition, London, Bailliere Tindall

Tolliss, D. (1995) Who was.. Down? *Nursing Times* 1st Feb 91(5): 61

Trotter, S. (2006) Cup feeding revisited. *MIDIRS Midwifery Digest* 16(3): 397–402

Trotter, S. (2008) Neonatal skin and cord care: implications for practice. Chapter 14. In: *Examination of Newborn and Neonatal Health: A Multidimensional Approach*. Davies, L., McDonald, S. (eds), Philadelphia, Churchill Livingstone Elsevier

Truman, P. (2006) Jaundice in the preterm infant. *Paediatric Nursing* 18(5): 20–22

UKNSPC (National Screening Programme Centre). (2007) *NHS Antenatal and Newborn Screening Programmes*. Online: http://www.newbornbloodspot. screening.nhs.uk

UK Newborn Screening Programme Centre (UKNSPC). (2008) *Standards and guidelines for newborn blood spot screening*. UK National Screening Committee. Online: http://www.newbornbloodspot.screening.nhs.uk

Ursell, B. (2005) Management of iron deficiency in pregnancy. *Midwives* 8(2): 78–79

References

Vennemann, M.M., Bajanowski, T., Brinkman, B., *et al*. The GeSID Study Group. (2009) Does breastfeeding reduce the risk of sudden infant death syndrome? *Pediatrics* 123(3): e406–e410

Ventolini, G., Samlowski, R., Hood, D.L. (2004) Placental findings in low-risk, singleton, term pregnancies after uncomplicated deliveries. *American Journal of Perinatology* 21(6): 325–328

Vergnano, S., Sharbind, M., Kazembe, P., Mwansambo, C., Heath, P. (2005) Neonatal sepsis: an international perspective. *Archives of Disease and Childhood: Fetal and Neonatal* 90(3): F220–F224

Victoria, C., Adair, L., Fall, C., *et al*. (2008) Maternal and child undernutrition: consequences for adult health and human capitol. *The Lancet* 371(9609): 340–357

Viles, R. (2007) Amniotic fluid embolism. Chapter 5. In: *The Confidential Enquiry into Maternal and Child Health (CEMACH) Saving Mothers' Lives: Reviewing Maternal Deaths to Make Motherhood Safer – 2003–2005*. The Seventh Report on Confidential Enquiries into Maternal Deaths in the UK. Lewis, G. (ed.), London, CEMACH

Vincent, M. (2003) Progress in a pocket. *Midwives* February 6(2): 82–84

Wallbank, S., Robertson, N. (2008) Midwife and nurse responses to miscarriage, stillbirth and neonatal death. *Evidence-based Midwifery* 6(3): 100–106

Ward, C., Mitchell, A. (2004) The experience of early motherhood –implications for care. *Evidence-based Midwifery* 2(1): 15–19

Warren, C. (2003) Why should I do vaginal examinations? In: *Midwifery Best Practice*, Wickham, S. (ed.), Edinburgh, Books for Midwives Press

Webster, J., Pritchard, M.A., Creedy, D., East, C. (2003) A simplified predictive index for the detection of women at risk for postnatal depression. *Birth* 30(2): 101–108

Wesnes, S.L., Rortveit, G., Bø, K.P.T., Hunskaar, S. (2007) Urinary incontinence during pregnancy. *Obstetrics and Gynecology* 109(4): 922–928

Westgren, M., Edvall, H., Nordstrom, E., Svalenius, E., Ranstam, J. (2005) Spontaneous cephalic version of breech presentation in the last trimester, *British Journal of Obstetrics and Gynaecology* 92(1): 19–22

Whitford, H.M., Alder, B., Jones, M. (2007) A longitudinal follow-up of women in their practice of perinatal pelvic floor exercises and stress urinary incontinence in North–East Scotland. *Midwifery* 23(3): 298–308

WHO (World Health Organisation). (2007) *Regional Office for Europe Health Evidence Network. Teenage Pregnancy Rates*. Online: http://www.euro.who.int/HEN

Williamson, A., Mullet, J., Bunting, M., Eason, J. (2005) Neonatal examination: are midwives clinically effective? *Midwives* 8(3): 116–118

Wills, G., Forster, D. (2008) Nausea and vomiting in pregnancy: what advice do midwives give? *Midwifery* 24(4): 390–398

Winterton Report. (1992) *Parliamentary Select Committee on Health. Second Report on the Maternity Services.* Vol. 2. London, HMSO

Wisborg, K., Kesmodel, U., Henriksen, T.B., *et al.* (2001) Exposure to tobacco smoke in utero and the risk of stillbirth and death in the first year of life. *American Journal of Epidemiology* 154(4): 322–327

Wright, A., Walker, J. (2007) Management of women who use drugs during pregnancy. *Seminars in Fetal and Neonatal Medicine* 12(2): 114–118

Yelland, J. (2010) Women's and midwives' views of early postnatal care. Chapter 3. In: *Essential Midwifery Practice: Postnatal Care.* Byrom, S., Edwards, G., Bick, D. (eds), Chichester, Wiley Blackwell